ABC of
Eating Disorders

ok is to ... ... p ... or before ... t date ...

WITHDRAWN

ABC series

The revised and updated ABC series – written by specialists for non-specialists

- With over 40 titles, this extensive series provides a quick and dependable reference on a broad range of topics in all the major specialities

- An easy-to-use resource, covering the symptoms, investigations, treatment and management of conditions presenting in your day-to-day practice

- Full colour photographs and illustrations aid diagnosis and patient understanding of a condition

- Each book in the new series now offers links to further information and articles, and a new dedicated website provides even more support

- A highly illustrated, informative and practical source of knowledge for GPs, GP registrars, junior doctors, doctors in training and those in primary care

For further information on the entire ABC series, please visit:

www.abcbookseries.com

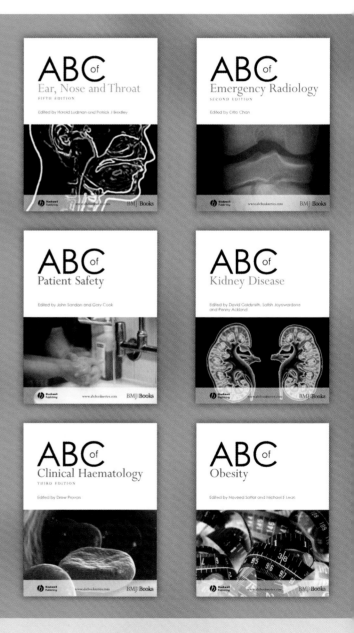

WILEY-BLACKWELL

BMJ|Books

ABC of

Eating Disorders

EDITED BY

Jane Morris

Consultant Psychiatrist
Child and Adolescent Mental Health Service
Royal Edinburgh Hospital
Edinburgh, UK

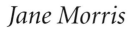 **WILEY-BLACKWELL**

A John Wiley & Sons, Ltd., Publication

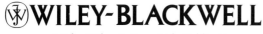 BMJ | Books

This edition first published 2008, © 2008 by Blackwell Publishing Ltd

BMJ Books is an imprint of BMJ Publishing Group Limited, used under licence by Blackwell Publishing which was acquired by John Wiley & Sons in February 2007. Blackwell's publishing programme has been merged with Wiley's global Scientific, Technical and Medical business to form Wiley-Blackwell.

Registered office: John Wiley & Sons Ltd, The Atrium, Southern Gate, Chichester, West Sussex, PO19 8SQ, UK

Editorial offices: 9600 Garsington Road, Oxford, OX4 2DQ, UK

The Atrium, Southern Gate, Chichester, West Sussex, PO19 8SQ, UK

111 River Street, Hoboken, NJ 07030–5774, USA

For details of our global editorial offices, for customer services and for information about how to apply for permission to reuse the copyright material in this book please see our website at www.wiley.com/wiley-blackwell

Library of Congress Cataloging-in-Publication Data

ABC of eating disorders / edited by Jane Morris.
     p. ; cm.
   Includes bibliographical references and index.
   ISBN 0-7279-1843-5
   1. Eating disorders. I. Morris, Jane, 1951-
   [DNLM: 1. Eating Disorders--Handbooks. WM 34 A134 2008]
   RC552.E18A23 2008
   616.85'26--dc22
                                        2007038358

ISBN: 978-0-7279-1843-7

A catalogue record for this book is available from the British Library.

Set in 9.25/12 pt Minion by Newgen Imaging Systems Pvt. Ltd, Chennai, India
Printed and bound in Singapore by COS Printers Pte Ltd

1   2008

Contents

Contributors

Jon Arcelus

Consultant Psychiatrist, Leicester Eating Disorders Service, Leicester General Hospital, Leicester, UK

Fiona Forbes

Consultant Psychiatrist, Child and Adolescent Mental Health Service, Royal Edinburgh Hospital, Edinburgh, UK

Nadine Harrison

General Practitioner, Richard Verney Medical Centre, University of Edinburgh, Edinburgh, UK

Ian MacDonald

Carer, Glasgow, UK

Heather Marrison

Former Service User, Edinburgh, UK

Brett McDermott

Associate Professor, Mater Child and Youth Mental Health Service, University of Queensland, South Brisbane, Australia

Jane Morris

Consultant Psychiatrist, Child and Adolescent Mental Health Service, Royal Edinburgh Hospital, Edinburgh, UK

Bob Palmer

Honorary Professor of Psychiatry, University of Leicester, and Consultant Psychiatrist, Leicester Eating Disorders Service, Leicester, UK

Glynis Read

Senior Therapist, Head of Training, Castle Craig Hospital, Blyth Bridge, Edinburgh, UK

Ulrike Schmidt

Professor of Eating Disorders, Section of Eating Disorders, Institute of Psychiatry, King's College London, London, UK

Grainne Smith

Carer and Writer, Stonehaven, UK

Anne Stewart

Consultant Adolescent Psychiatrist, Oxfordshire and Buckinghamshire Mental Health Partnership NHS Trust and Honorary Senior Lecturer, University of Oxford, Oxford, UK

Rosemary Stewart

Carer and Counsellor, Edinburgh, UK

Jacinta Tan

Senior Clinical Research Fellow and Honorary Consultant Child and Adolescent Psychiatrist, The Ethox Centre, University of Oxford, Oxford, UK

Janet Treasure

Professor, Department of Academic Psychiatry, King's College London, London, UK

Chris Williams

Senior Lecturer in Psychiatry and Honorary Consultant Psychiatrist, NHS Greater Glasgow and Clyde Psychological Medicine, Gartnavel Royal Hospital, Glasgow, UK

Geoffrey Wolff

Consultant Psychiatrist, Gerald Russell Eating Disorders Unit, South London and Maudsley NHS Foundation Trust, London, UK

Alex Yellowlees

Consultant Psychiatrist, Medical Director, Priory Hospital, Glasgow, UK

Preface

A few years ago we wondered why on earth there was no *ABC of Eating Disorders* in the well-known series. Accessible paperbacks and websites are devoured avidly by patients and their families, and there is no lack of scholarly works by and for specialists. General practitioners frequently find themselves less knowledgeable than the patients or parents so desperate for their help—or so self-destructively avoiding it. General psychiatrists have focussed their expertise on psychoses and depressive disorders, with the result that a general adult psychiatric ward can be the most dangerous place to admit someone with anorexia nervosa. Meanwhile hospital physicians and nurses find it hard to tolerate the apparent self-destructiveness.

There was clearly a need for basic primer for doctors, spanning but differentiating *A*norexia and *B*ulimia nervosa and *C*hildhood eating disorders. In fact we have aimed the text at professional readers of all disciplines who work with eating disorders—either as a primary diagnosis or arising in the course of something else. Many lay carers and sufferers themselves will be able to read and appreciate the information. It may still have something to teach those embarking on specialist eating disorders careers but the primary aim is general practitioners and their colleagues in the community who—more than ever—need to incorporate a sophisticated awareness of this field into their professional practice.

It was naïve, though, to think that meeting such an obvious need would be straightforward. Like many of my young patients, this book has had to survive a series of transitions. Particular thanks to Eleanor Lines of BMJ Books for her enthusiasm and refusal to let me give up, and to Mary Banks and Adam Gilbert at Blackwell Publishing for taking over, taking care to preserve what was good and encouraging me to expand the scope of the book from a 'picture book' to a more authoritative account.

It is certainly still an ABC—informing a compassionate *A*ttitude, understanding *B*ackground causes and formulating effective *C*aring strategies. I have become steadily more convinced, though, that 'Eating Disorders' is an unhelpful misnomer for conditions whose roots are merely reflected in eating—as well as other—behaviours, and which certainly do not respond to treatments aimed in a blinkered way at 'correcting' weight and eating.

I am grateful to authors and co-authors for their generous response and for burning midnight oil to write to deadlines after their long day jobs. And to Alice Nelson who has miraculously helped us all meet the deadlines. Particular thanks to the sufferers and carers who agreed to revisit painful memories and to write frankly about them—I resisted suggestions that we might tone down criticisms of our profession. However, it is to our wonderful medical students—particularly those who aspire to General Practice—that I should like to dedicate the *ABC of Eating Disorders*, in the hope and faith that a future generation of doctors will be able to offer a more intelligent and compassionate approach.

Jane Morris

CHAPTER 1

Diagnosis of Eating Disorders

Jane Morris

OVERVIEW

- 'Eating disorders' is a misnomer for obsessive weight-losing disorders ('anorexia nervosa') and other body image-related disorders ('bulimia nervosa' and 'binge eating disorder').
- Sufferers value weight loss, and see their weight-losing behaviour as essential to avoid fatness. A sympathetic climate of awareness is essential for diagnosis.
- At low weight, the physical and psychological consequences of starvation amplify the obsessive drive for thinness and cause risk to life.
- At low weight physical risk results from impaired resistance to infection, self-poisoning (accidental or deliberate), electrolytic instability and damage to heart muscle.
- Quality of life can be improved long-term by diagnosing eating disorders and remaining engaged so that risk can be managed during the long recovery process.

Box 1.1 **Mortality in eating disorders**

Sten Theander's early follow-up studies found that a shocking 20% of anorexic patients died of causes related to the disorder. Even now, mortality in anorexia nervosa is 10 times that in the general population and is among the top three or four causes of death in teenagers. Today's lower mortality figures partly reflect changes in diagnostic criteria—we now require only 15% body weight to be lost before making the diagnosis (or BMI below 17.5) compared with 25% (BMI below 15).

Improved management may also contribute to more favourable longevity—it is now acknowledged that a tolerant, respectful relationship allows long-term physical monitoring and support to be offered during the years it often takes for patients to summon the motivational strength to overcome their obsessive weight-losing behaviour. A significant minority do not fully recover but are at least enabled to live valuable or tolerable lives.

Some deaths result from ambivalently-taken overdoses that would not have killed healthy weight individuals. Although starvation almost inevitably results in depression, we cannot conclude that all these 'suicides' were intended as such. Likewise, the effects of substance abuse are greatly amplified at low weight. The majority of deaths occur in winter months: hypothermia, infections (including tuberculosis) and organ failure account for many more fatalities. The starved heart is especially vulnerable when overexercised.

Most people occasionally experience disordered eating, and resolve to be more restrained. Women—who make up 90% of sufferers from eating disorders—especially struggle between appetite and food adverts on one hand, and the dictates of fashion designers and warnings of obesity experts on the other. Ten per cent of teenage girls induce vomiting from time to time, and 4% of young women will develop a significant eating disorder during their life. How can we distinguish between transient disordered eating and more lasting problems that damage health—and, in the extreme, threaten life itself (Box 1.1)?

Eating behaviours span a range of body weights, behavioural and psychological disturbances (Figure 1.1). There are core diagnostic criteria for anorexia nervosa (AN) (Box 1.2), bulimia nervosa (BN) (Box 1.3) and—most recently—for binge eating disorder (BED). Patients should be treated according to the 'best fit' of symptoms.

What are 'eating disorders'?

In fact eating is not the only disordered behaviour in what might be better thought of as 'weight-losing disorders'. Self-starvation,

self-induced vomiting, compulsive activity and exercise, use of laxatives, diet pills, herbal medicines and deliberate exposure to the cold are some of the behaviours seen in the pursuit of thinness. For the majority of eating disordered people today, the pursuit of thinness seems like a culturally endorsed solution to life's difficulties and a route to better self-esteem (Box 1.4). For the minority with low weight AN, cultural factors coexist with a predisposition to experience satisfaction or relief as a result of weight loss. This 'addiction' to self-starvation can exist even in the absence of cultural approval of thinness.

What is anorexia nervosa?

The core feature of AN is deliberate weight loss, with fear of weight gain, and a problem of body image which translates all the patient's distress into a perception that their body is too fat. To meet

ABC of Eating Disorders. Edited by J. Morris. © 2008 Blackwell Publishing, ISBN: 978-0-7279-1843-7.

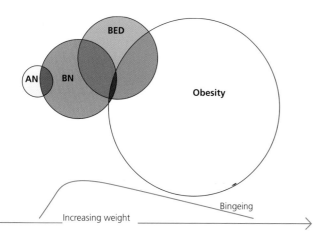

Figure 1.1 Sufferers from anorexia nervosa (AN) make up only a small minority of patients with eating disorders. There is some diagnostic overlap with bulimia nervosa (BN) in that about 50% 'graduate' to binge-purge disorders with gradually rising weight. Normal weight BN involves the most extreme binges because of the purge behaviours which result in 'binge-priming'. When purging does not occur, in binge eating disorder (BED), binges tend to be smaller but weight is often higher and may be in the overweight or obese range. So-called 'simple obesity' occurs when overeating is more general rather than characterized by discrete 'binges', and body image concern is more likely to be a secondary result rather than the root cause of the overeating.

Box 1.2 DSM-IV criteria for anorexia nervosa

A Refusal to maintain body weight at or above a minimally normal weight for age and height (e.g. weight loss leading to maintenance of body weight less than 85% of that expected or failure to make expected weight gain during period of growth, leading to body weight less than 85% of that expected).

B Intense fear of gaining weight or becoming fat, even though underweight.

C Disturbance in the way in which one's body weight or shape is experienced, undue influence of body weight or shape on self-evaluation, or denial of the seriousness of the current low body weight.

D In postmenarchal females, amenorrhoea, i.e. the absence of at least three consecutive menstrual cycles.

Box 1.3 DSM-IV criteria for bulimia nervosa

A Recurrent episodes of binge-eating, characterized by the following:
- eating in a discrete period of time (e.g. a 2-hour period) an amount of food that is definitely larger than most people would eat during a similar period of time and similar circumstances.
- a sense of lack of control during the episode.

B Recurrent inappropriate compensatory behaviour in order to prevent weight gain, such as self-induced vomiting, misuse of laxatives, diuretics, other medications or enemas.

C The binge-eating and compensatory behaviours occur on average at least twice a week for 3 months.

D Self-evaluation is unduly influenced by body weight and shape.

E The disturbance does not occur exclusively during episodes of anorexia nervosa.

Box 1.4 Eating disorders in ethnic and cultural minorities

- Wilful starvation may not be associated with an overvaluation of weight and shape even in Westernized families.
- For some patients—particularly devout young Muslim girls—an association with religion may be apparent, with starvation-induced obsessionality dictating many extra prayer rituals, and with fasting carrying religious rather than 'slimming' overtones.
- Community religious advisors can help discriminate between culturally appropriate dietary restriction and obsessionality.
- People of West Indian and African origins tend to be less vulnerable culturally to eating disorders—they are better able to relish a voluptuous figure, and also carry distressing associations of thinness with emaciation and acquired immunodeficiency syndrome (AIDS)—for such people a thin body may be heavily stigmatized.
- The Curacao study found that even in 'fat-admiring' cultures there is a small, core prevalence of anorexia nervosa. However, more culturally sensitive bulimic disorders may occur far less.

---

diagnostic criteria, at least 15% of minimum normal weight must have been lost. For adults, this means body mass index (BMI) is below 17.5. Menstruation is absent (though women who take the contraceptive pill have withdrawal bleeds). In males low testosterone causes atrophied genitalia and absence of morning erections.

Some people with AN maintain low weight by starvation alone, or starvation plus exercising—this is 'restrictive' AN. In the more dangerous 'binge-purge' subtype, the sufferer induces vomiting or takes laxatives, diuretics or 'slimming pills' in an attempt to get rid of calories. 'Binges' are usually much smaller than in BN.

What is bulimia nervosa?

Bulimia nervosa is characterized by dietary restriction, followed by breakthrough 'binges' then purging behaviours. This sets up a vicious circle in which binges become larger—often involving thousands of calories in a single binge—and normal social life is disrupted. Binges are not simply large snacks, but a qualitatively different experience in which control is lost and foods normally avoided are guiltily consumed. Binge-purge episodes become a learned response to all stress.

By definition, people with BN have a BMI in the normal range (or above).

What is binge eating disorder?

Binge eating disorder was formerly known as 'non-purging bulimia'. Binges occur without compensatory behaviours such as purging, fasting or exercise. Patients are more likely to be overweight or obese and are torn between the desire to restrain their eating to lose weight and the opposing wish to stabilize their eating habits and thus their lives.

How often is a general practitioner likely to encounter an eating disorder?

The average list is likely to include two or three patients with serious AN, 15–20 with chronic BN, and many more with BED. Figures are higher in student health centres and practices serving younger people.

Why make a diagnosis?

Making a positive diagnosis of an eating disorder saves fruitless investigation and treatment. Anorexia nervosa is the commonest cause of significant weight loss in adolescents. It is important not to overlook diabetes, thyrotoxicosis, cystic fibrosis or other causes of weight loss, but in practice young people often undergo extensive investigations while their eating disorder is neglected.

The distinction between AN and BN is particularly important. Standard treatments for BN are ineffective against low weight binge-purge disorders, and physical danger is high. Purging behaviours at low weight increase mortality greatly, particularly if alcohol or other substance abuse is involved. On the other hand, normal weight BN, though distressing and damaging, is associated with little increase in mortality, and has a better prognosis when managed with evidence-based treatments.

Picking up eating disorders—a climate of awareness

Patients with AN may be 'brought' to the doctor by worried parents, and do better with early treatment. Bulimia nervosa and BED are more secret, with an average of 6 years from onset to presentation. In adults, longer duration of BN is associated with better prognosis once treatment starts, but there is growing evidence that early diagnosis of BN, in adolescence, provides a window of opportunity for interrupting the vicious circle before it becomes chronic. There is concern that 'binge-priming' behaviours in the young, such as dieting, purging and other weight-losing behaviours may not only predispose to later BN, but also to substance abuse of various sorts.

The key to recognizing secret eating disorders—like alcohol problems—is to make a habit of anticipating the possibility. It is a good habit to routinely ask young female patients about their eating habits. The SCOFF questionnaire (Box 1.5) is a validated brief instrument to screen for eating disorders, similar in concept to the CAGE questionnaire for alcohol problems.

Box 1.5 SCOFF questionnaire (Morgan *et al.* 1999)

- Do you make yourself **S**ick because you feel uncomfortably full?
- Do you worry you have lost **C**ontrol over how much you eat?
- Have you recently lost more than **O**ne stone (6 kg) in weight over a 3-month period?
- Do you believe yourself to be **F**at when others say you are thin?
- Would you say that **F**ood dominates your life?

Women complaining of menstrual irregularities or fertility problems should be screened for eating disorders. Unexplained seizures, funny turns, and chronic fatigue should also prompt the consideration. Sometimes gastrointestinal complaints are both the consequence of and the 'cover' for eating disorders. More 'psychological' presentations include depression, anxiety, obsessional symptoms and problems with relationships or at school/work. Bulimia nervosa

is often diagnosed by dentists (vomiting affects tooth enamel) and occasionally by police, if binges lead to shoplifting.

Male sufferers are particularly unlikely to be diagnosed and helped, so that while females are clearly at higher risk, any male patient with unexplained weight loss should be asked about dietary and exercise habits.

Making a diagnosis, not an accusation

Eating disorders may be secret, shame-ridden and even dangerous, but they are misfortunes not crimes. It is important to ask sympathetic, matter-of-fact questions, not to sound accusing. Treatment is then more likely to be accepted as help, rather than resisted as punishment.

Forging and keeping a helpful relationship with eating disorder patients

Eating disorders begin as solutions to difficulties. In chronic cases, AN becomes an identity. Even when patients realize their 'solution' causes problems, they remain ambivalent. Attempts to 'frighten' patients out of the disorder may only increase their habitual anxiety-reducing strategies—starvation and binge-purging! Attempts to bulldoze resistance find the patient staunchly defending their eating disorder.

Those who explore ambivalence sensitively, seeking to understand both pros and cons of the eating disorder, are more likely to find themselves on the side of the patient *against* the disorder. Patients find it less daunting to give up their eating disorder if they can learn alternative coping skills.

When AN acutely threatens life we are obliged to take action, but when patients are not in extremis, the priority is to maintain useful contact, and keep the door open for them to accept as much help as possible. Medical monitoring, and a listening ear, keep hope—and patients—alive. Recent studies show that recovery is still possible 20 years after the onset of AN.

Essentials of assessment

It is essential to measure and weigh patients, to calculate BMI (Box 1.6). Even specialists cannot estimate this accurately by eye. Body mass index distinguishes AN from other eating disorders, and provides a baseline for monitoring trends in weight change. For children and young teenagers, BMI is plotted on centile charts against age.

Box 1.6 Equation for Quatelet's body mass index (BMI)

$$BMI = \frac{\text{weight in kilograms}}{(\text{height in metres})^2}$$

If there is weight loss, ask when this started, and what was happening then? Document the patient's highest and lowest weights, preferred weight, and the range s/he would accept. Get an idea of current daily food intake, and patterns of purging and exercise, alcohol, drugs and medication. For patients with a BMI below 14 or a precipitous decline in weight (>1 kg/week), mortality is greatly increased by purging and by comorbid substance abuse. Such patients should be urgently discussed with specialists. Some need medical admission, using a section of the Mental Health Act if necessary to save life.

Particular danger signs in emaciated patients are weakness (unable to climb stairs or to rise from a squat), chest pain and cognitive slowing. Admission for rest, warmth, rehydration and medical monitoring can save life, particularly when it is cold—most deaths occur in winter. However, medical wards often struggle without support from eating disorders specialists. General psychiatric wards may be the most dangerous places of all, although suicidal anorexic patients may need to be managed here. There should be a low threshold of suspicion for the investigation and management of overdoses. These prove fatal more readily in emaciated people.

Responsible investigation

When a patient is in extremis, outpatient investigations waste time and expose vulnerable individuals to cold, infection and unnecessary exertion. In safer circumstances blood tests maintain contact with patients and demonstrate that your concern extends beyond the number on the scales. Biochemistry, with glucose and thyroid levels, usefully excludes some differential diagnoses. Glucose is low in AN (unless there is coexistent poorly controlled diabetes). The thyroid may be underactive in AN, and it is unwise to endanger the heart by prescribing thyroxine. Electrolytes may show low urea (reflecting protein intake), and low potassium (vomiting). Liver function tests may suggest comorbid drug or alcohol problems, though extreme starvation alone causes liver damage.

Anorexia nervosa usually causes anaemia, and if white count is *not* low infection is likely. Raised mean corpuscular volume (MCV) suggests alcohol problems.

Electrocardiograms (ECGs) provide immediate, sensitive reflexions of electrolyte and cardiac status. Chest X-rays can reveal infections as well as rib fractures. After a year or more at low weight a dual energy X-ray absorptiometry (DEXA) bone scan provides a useful perspective on the risk of osteoporosis.

Remember pregnancy tests and contraceptive advice. Even at unhealthily low weight, women may become pregnant, and vomiting makes oral contraception unreliable.

Always assess mood—the risk of suicide is raised in people with eating disorders. Self-rated questionnaires can be useful tools for tracking changes in mood and eating disordered attitudes, and help patients to collaborate in evaluating their symptoms (see Further resources, below). Consideration of psychological state is a helpful way to find common ground with patients who reject physical concerns.

Further reading

American Psychiatric Association. *Diagnostic and Statistical Manual of Mental Disorders*, 4th edn. American Psychiatric Association, Washington, D.C., 1994.

Birmingham CL & Beumont PJV, eds. *Medical Management of Eating Disorders: A Practical Handbook for Healthcare Professionals*. Cambridge University Press, Cambridge, 2004.

Fairburn, C. *Overcoming Binge Eating*. Guilford Press, New York, 1995. (*A very readable classic of self-help whose introductory first half provides an essential background to the evidence base for BN, even though it is now a little out of date.*)

Hoek HW. Incidence, prevalence and mortality of anorexia nervosa and other eating disorders. *Current Opinions in Psychiatry* 2006; **19**: 389–394.

NICE. *Eating Disorders: Core Interventions in the Treatment and Management of Anorexia Nervosa, Bulimia Nervosa and Related Eating Disorders*. NICE Clinical Guideline No 9. National Institute for Clinical Excellence, London, 2004: http://www.nice.org.uk (*The website is particularly useful in comprising a quick reference version and also a users' and carers' version of the Guideline.*)

Treasure J. *Breaking Free from Anorexia Nervosa: A Survival Guide for Families, Friends and Sufferers*. Psychology Press, Hove, 1997. (*An accessible text conveying essential information in a readable and therapeutic style— recommended for professionals as much as for patients.*)

Further resources: list of useful questionnaires and rating scales

Eating Disorders Examination—self-report version (EDE-Q)

The gold standard eating disorders questionnaire in the self-report version. This covers a range of anorexic behaviours including eating.

Fairburn CG & Beglin SJ. Assessment of eating disorders: interview or self-report questionnaire? *International Journal of Eating Disorders* 1994; **16**: 363–370.

Fairburn CG & Cooper Z. The eating disorder examination. In: Fairburn CG & Wilson GT, eds. *Binge Eating: Nature, Assessment, and Treatment*. Guilford Press, New York, 1993: 317–360.

The Bulimic Investigatory Test, Edinburgh (BITE)

Henderson M & Freeman CPL. A self-rating scale for bulimia. The BITE. *British Journal of Psychiatry* 1987; **150**: 18–24.

The Beck Depression Inventory (BDI)

Beck AT, Ward C & Mendelson M. An inventory for measuring depression. *Archives of General Psychiatry* 1961; **4**: 561–585.

The second edition (BDI-II) is a more sophisticated version—but beware, most depression rating scales include items on appetite and weight change, which will not reflect mood helpfully in the presence of an eating disorder.

CHAPTER 2

Causes of Eating Disorders

Bob Palmer

OVERVIEW

- The precise pathogenesis of eating disorders remains uncertain.
- There is a widely held belief that social pressures to slim are the most important cause of eating disorders. However, other factors must be involved.
- These may include genetic and psychosocial factors.
- Most of the psychosocial factors are non-specific and have been shown to be relevant also to other mental disorders.
- Beliefs about causation may affect the attitude to treatments of both patient and clinician.

Knowing the cause of a disorder may or may not be of help in treatment. Furthermore, what starts a disorder may not be what maintains it, and the latter may be of greater practical importance. The prominent cognitive-behavioural models of eating disorders (EDs) focus mainly upon how to overcome maintaining factors. However, ideas about causation may affect our attitudes and crucially those of our patients and those who care for and about them.

Popular certainty

It is no surprise that nowadays most people know something about the characteristics of EDs. What is perhaps more surprising is that many people feel they know what causes them. Few would claim with similar conviction to know the causes of leukaemia or ulcerative colitis or ingrowing toenails. Anorexia nervosa (AN) and bulimia nervosa (BN) are different. They seem to be *about* something and that 'something' has to do with personal and social pressures of which we are all aware to some degree. Surely, many suggest, the grim self-starvation and hatred of fat of the person with AN must have some relationship with the commonplace behaviour of slimming that is within the experience of nearly everyone. And many believe that this in turn must be linked with the way in which being slim—sometimes nearly emaciated—is held up as being the ideal for both health and beauty. Likewise, surely binge eating

represents an exaggeration of the self-indulgence which again is a part of most people's experience. It all seems self-evident. We blame the media. We tut-tut about the decadence of modern society. Secretly and self-righteously we entertain the thought that anyone who lets these forces influence them to the extent of making them ill must be rather silly. Even more secretly, we may experience a smidgeon of admiration for the self-control which the person with AN achieves when many of us feel lacking in that respect. Hence, the hackneyed response trotted out at social gatherings, 'Oh, anorexia nervosa, I could do with a bit of that'. Such comments are a pale echo of the 'pro-ana' and 'pro-mia' websites which advocate the idea that EDs are to be thought of as lifestyle choices rather than disorders, an interpretation that seems to ride roughshod over the way in which the conditions at best shrink the experience and autonomy of the sufferer and at worst lead to death.

Expert uncertainty

The literature on EDs, scientific and popular, may share the convictions of the general public. However, sometimes other causes are cited with similar vehemence. They range from zinc deficiency through brain abnormalities and developmental problems to the contradictions inherent in the role of women in late capitalist society. With so many theories, canny observers are likely to conclude that none is adequate and decide that for the present we cannot be sure about what causes EDs. Nevertheless, something can be said about aetiology even if it does not yet amount to a satisfactory account. And some of the things that can be said may have useful implications for the clinician. However, an open mind is required.

The following is a brief account of the more important factors that are probably involved in the genesis and perpetuation of EDs. It will concentrate upon issues that may have relevance to the clinician. Most factors will get a mention although they are not arranged into a coherent aetiological theory; it is as Eric Morecombe once said of his piano playing, 'all the right notes are there but not necessarily in the right order'.

Eating restraint

Firstly, slimming is relevant. It does seem that 'eating restraint'—the general term used by psychologists for voluntary

---

ABC of Eating Disorders. Edited by J. Morris. © 2008 Blackwell Publishing, ISBN: 978-0-7279-1843-7.

Box 2.1 **Some effects of eating restraint**

• Increased drive to eat
• Preoccupation with thoughts of food and eating
• Increased sensitivity to external cues about eating
• Tendency to eat more still having eaten more than original intention ('counterregulation')
• Tendency to binge eat
• Tendency to be emotional

Box 2.2 **The Minnesota starvation experiment**

As the Second World War was ending, starvation was widespread in Europe. Dr Ancel Keys and his collaborators conducted a study which aimed to explore the effects of starvation and the best methods of refeeding.

Thirty-six men volunteered. They were mainly conscientious objectors to military service. They were selected as being both physically and mentally fit.

After 3 months of initial observation, the men were fed a diet of about 1600 Kcal per day which was less than half their usual baseline intake. They lost about a quarter of their body weight. After 6 months on the 'semi-starvation' regime, they were refed in various ways back to their former weight.

Thirty-two men completed the experiment. Most of the men experienced most of the features listed in Box 2.1 together with lethargy, tiredness and a variety of physical symptoms. Mental changes were prominent and included notable preoccupation with food and eating which for some lasted long after the end of the experiment.

The primary two-volume account of the experiment, *The Biology of Human Starvation* (Keys *et al*. 1950), is difficult to obtain. A lay summary and discussion may be found in the recent book *Hunger; an Unnatural History* (Russell 2005).

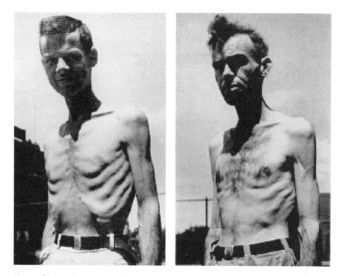

Figure 2.1 Volunteers in the Minnesota experiments. *Life* magazine photograph of conscientious objectors during starvation experiment (30 July 1945, **19**(5), p. 43). (Credit: Wallace Kirkland/Time Life Pictures/Getty Images)

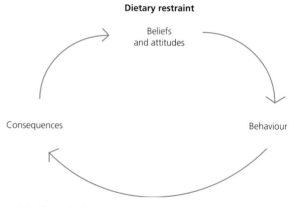

Figure 2.2 The cycle of restraint.

undereating in the presence of an intact appetite—plays some part in the stories of most people who develop EDs. This goes for BN as well as AN.

The consequences of eating restraint upon the experience and behaviour of the person have been extensively studied and the key features are summarized in Box 2.1. The classic demonstration remains the Minnesota starvation study of over 60 years ago in which male conscientious objectors volunteered to undergo a regime of semi-starvation for 9 months (Box 2.2; Figure 2.1). The Minnesota subjects showed many of the features of people with EDs despite their gender and having been selected for their mental health.

Eating restraint is a motivated behaviour with consequences. If those consequences tend to increase the motivation then there is the possibility of a vicious circle (Figure 2.2). The more heightened the consequences, the greater the risk of their tending to increase the motivation to restrain through fear of the perceived catastrophe of letting go and 'losing control'. Such positive feedback and the ensuing vicious circle may plausibly play a significant part in the genesis of the main EDs. The implication for the clinician is that helping the patient to eat regularly and substantially may not

only correct any weight deficit but might also tend to quench the consequences of restraint and unwind the vicious circle.

Many but not all subjects start their ED career with restraint that is motivated by apparently commonplace ideas about wishing to be slimmer and/or the fear of becoming 'fat'. Coming from a family where such issues are emphasized increases the risk. However, what might be called the weight, shape and slimming zeitgeist cannot explain everything, because whilst such 'pressures' are almost by definition widespread, especially in the lives of young women, only a few—perhaps 2 or 3%—fall ill with an ED. The slimming culture may operate by recruiting the many into embarking upon eating restraint. But what makes the few so vulnerable that they go on to develop a clinical ED?

Biological vulnerability

Established EDs have physical components, although most are likely to be consequences rather than antecedents. However, some

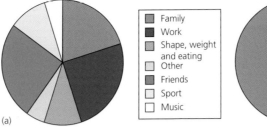

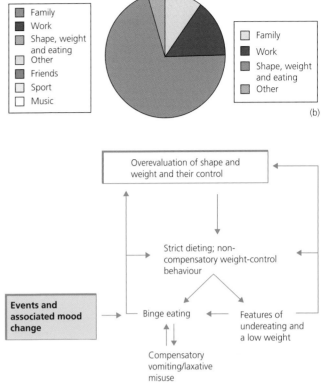

Figure 2.3 Transdiagnostic diagram.
(a) A 'balanced' pie chart. (b) An 'unbalanced'
pie chart. (Adapted from Fairburn 2008)

(a)

(b)

may be causally relevant. For instance, there is evidence that birth trauma and prematurity increase the risk of AN and that this could be the background to some of the abnormalities—both structural and functional—that have been found using brain imaging techniques. Studies of early-onset AN reveal unilateral hypoperfusion in the temporal lobe which does not vary with nutrition, although the more frequently observed sulcal widening and ventricular enlargement may well be a consequence of the disorder rather than a risk factor.

Over the last couple of decades there has been confirmation that EDs tend to run in families and do so in a manner that suggests genetic transmission. So the hunt is on for relevant genes but without clear results so far. Indeed, it seems unlikely that there would be just one gene that was associated with the vulnerability to any or all of the EDs. It is more likely that risk is influenced by many genes each of small effect in this respect. It is a matter of speculation what might be the phenotype of relevant genes. Indeed, some may code for some hidden internal differences ('endophenotypes'). Other more psychological features that may be biologically underpinned include obsessionality, perfectionism and a cognitive rigidity detectable as difficulty with set shifting.

Studies of neurotransmitters and hormones often find differences between ED samples and the comparison groups. However, the significance and implications of the findings are unclear. The pharmaceutical industry is investing in drugs affecting eating but their concern is with obesity rather than EDs. Perhaps some crumbs may fall from that table. For the present, the only drug treatment with an evidence base remains the use of antidepressants in BN and the beneficial effects are modest.

Psychosocial vulnerability

Between the ubiquitous social influences and the possibility of particular genetic and biological risk factors lies the psychosocial domain. It is here that the observations of clinicians and clinical researchers are most fruitful. Their observations suggest that EDs share with other psychiatric disorders a raft of characteristics that may be risk factors. Thus before or as they develop their disorders, people who come to have ED tend to be stressed and unhappy. Compared to non-clinical comparison groups, they report having experienced more abuse and more adversity in general. Furthermore, they have notably low self-esteem. What is more specific to people with EDs is that by the time that they develop their disorder such self-worth as they have tends to be invested largely in the precarious stock of their ability to control their body weight and shape (Figure 2.3). Their wider problems have become entangled with

Figure 2.4 The transdiagnostic 'template' formulation. (Adapted from Fairburn 2008)

ideas about weight and eating in a way that far exceeds the normative weight concern that means that most of us would feel that life might be a bit better if we were half a stone lighter.

Models

Just how an ED comes about and is perpetuated remains uncertain although it is possible—and often useful—to draw models of the box and arrow type. Thus Fairburn and colleagues have proposed a model which they describe as 'transdiagnostic' and applicable to all EDs (Figure 2.4). Such formulations tend to emphasize perpetuation rather than origination. Adapted for and with the individual, they provide a useful basis for conversation with the patient in psychological treatment.

Implications

Both the patient and the clinician may be influenced in their attitudes to the task of change by their ideas about causation and the nature of EDs. The clinician needs to assess the motives that drive the eating restraint and develop ideas—a story—about the patient's particular psychological problems and how the two issues may be entangled. General ideas about risk factors and so on need to be used in an open-minded way to illuminate the particular case. Furthermore, in the age of the internet, clinicians need to be able to make sensible responses to the undigested 'facts' and opinions delivered by their patients' latest Google search. We need to keep a balance between our necessary scepticism and our patients' need for us to show therapeutic enthusiasm.

Further reading

Fairburn CG. *Cognitive Behaviour Therapy for Eating Disorders.* Guilford Press, New York, 2008.

Fairburn CG, Welch SL, Doll HA *et al.* Risk factors for bulimia nervosa; a community based case-controlled study. *Archives of General Psychiatry* 1997; **4**: 509–517.

Keys A, Brozek J, Henschel A, Mickelson O & Taylor HL. *The Biology of Human Starvation.* University of Minnesota Press, Minneapolis, 1950.

Palmer RL. Concepts of eating disorders. In: Treasure J, Schmidt U, Dare C & Van Furth E, eds. *Handbook of Eating Disorders*, 2nd edn. John Wiley & Sons, Chichester, 2003: 1–10.

Russell SA. *Hunger; an Unnatural History.* Basic Books, New York, 2005.

Strober M & Bulik C. Genetic epidemiology of eating disorders. In: Fairburn CG & Brownell KD, eds. *Eating Disorders and Obesity; a Comprehensive Handbook*, 2nd edn, 2002: 238–242.

CHAPTER 3

Body Image Disturbance in Eating Disorders

Glynis Read and Jane Morris

OVERVIEW

- Body image distress is usually (though not invariably) the driving force for the onset and maintenance of eating disorders.
- The construct 'body image' is more complex than often believed and includes a range of dimensions, which may need to be specifically addressed.
- Improvement in terms of weight and eating disorder behaviours may mask continuing body image distress.
- Body image acceptance is important for lasting recovery.
- Specific treatment to promote body image acceptance is rarely provided even in specialist eating disorder services, leaving apparently recovered sufferers at increased risk of relapse.
- High levels of self-esteem may allow individuals to set body image concerns in a healthier perspective, and interventions promoting healthy self-esteem may act as preventative measures against eating disorders in schools and colleges, even without specifically addressing body image.

The importance of body image in eating disorders

Extreme body image concern is recognized as a precursor for eating disorders in at risk populations and as the main factor in the psychopathology of eating disorders (Box 3.1). Disordered eating is used by many as a way of improving body image, in the quest for better self-esteem. Indeed an eating disorder may represent a 'false solution' for improving a negative body image. The challenge is to come to terms with body image without using eating disorder pathology to sort it out.

Body image acceptance has been shown to be crucial in lasting recovery from eating disorders (Garner 2004), yet remarkably little emphasis has been placed on body image in therapy.

The previous chapter addressed the multiple causes of eating disorders. Historically and geographically distant cases of anorexia nervosa (AN) have been observed with religious or commercial roots, but in present day prosperous countries extreme weight and

Box 3.1 **Case vignette: Amanda**

As a teenager Amanda had low weight anorexia nervosa but managed to avoid contact with services. In her 20s she finally sought treatment because her weight was rising very much against her will. To her great distress she found herself bingeing at the end of each day, and ended up inducing vomiting. This resulted in further loss of control and continuing weight gain. She was so horrified by her new plump body that she wore dark baggy clothes even in summer and grew her hair long over her face to conceal her 'fat' cheeks. She dropped out of college and quit her part-time job.

She noticed people giving her curious looks and was convinced they were disgusted by her size. She stayed in the house to avoid scrutiny, but as a result found herself spending more and more time eating. It proved impossible for her to attend therapy sessions by daylight until her mother offered to pay for a counsellor to visit her flat.

shape concern is the driving force for most eating disorders and influences long-term outcome. Negative body image is a diagnostic criterion for AN and bulimia nervosa (BN) in both main psychiatric diagnostic classifications (Table 3.1). Binge eaters also suffer

Table 3.1 Formal body image criteria for anorexia nervosa and bulimia nervosa. (From Cash & Pruzinsky 2004, p. 470)

	ICD 10 (WHO 1992)	DSM-IV (APA 2000)
Anorexia nervosa	There is body-image distortion in the form of a specific psychopathology whereby a dread of fatness persists as an intrusive, overvalued idea and the patient imposes a low weight threshold on himself or herself	Disturbance in the way in which one's body weight or shape is experienced, undue influence of body weight or shape on self-evaluation, or denial of the seriousness of the current low body weight
Bulimia nervosa	The psychopathology consists of a morbid dread of fatness and the patient sets herself or himself a sharply defined weight threshold, well below the premorbid weight that constitutes the optimum or healthy weight in the opinion of the physician	Self-evaluation is unduly influenced by body shape and weight

ABC of Eating Disorders. Edited by J. Morris. © 2008 Blackwell Publishing, ISBN: 978-0-7279-1843-7.

from negative body image (Marcus *et al.* 1992) although it is not formalized as a diagnostic criterion.

Physically and behaviourally 'successful' treatment may not bring body image satisfaction. Greater change has been reported in questionnaires for eating behaviours than for body image. Follow-up studies suggest that body disparagement causes significant distress in people who have restored body weight and eating patterns, and the level of body image distress at the end of treatment predicts relapse. The risk of relapse may be enhanced because of inadequate provision of treatment for extreme shape and weight concern within most currently offered eating disorder treatment.

Understanding the concept of body image

The concept of body image is complex and multifaceted. It refers to an individual's view of their body size, shape, weight and appearance, and may focus either on the body as a whole or on specific parts. The term integrates values and judgements which may vary along different dimensions in different individuals. Body weight, measurements, shape and texture of flesh ('muscular' versus 'flabby') may all be involved.

The complex body image construct may be considered to include four main components:
- *perceptual distortion*—visual or tactile illusions leading to misjudgement of the true size or shape of the body or its parts;
- *body dissatisfaction*—a feeling or judgment about the body, regardless of how accurately it is perceived;
- *behaviours*—reflecting the individual's beliefs and concerns about their body image;
- *cognitions*—the thoughts, assumptions and beliefs held by the individual about their body image in the context of their lives.

These components all interact with each other as represented in Figure 3.1.

The nature of the perceptual disturbance

Perceptual distortion may take the form of an imagined bodily defect or exaggeration of features in which a discrepancy occurs between actual and perceived size. Studies show that this misperception does not occur at the level of sensory deficits (Farrell *et al.* 2005). Shafran & Robinson (2004) have suggested a mechanism which they call 'thought-shape fusion'. For example, an anorexic patient who 'feels' fat comes to believes she must therefore appear fat to others. This may go so far as a person fearing that even thinking or dreaming about food will make them fat. Such superstitious, 'magical' thinking is similar to thinking styles seen in obsessive compulsive disorder (OCD).

Overestimation of size is further amplified by a combination of behaviours such as body checking and selective attention to, or avoidance of, certain body parts. This is precisely the sort of behaviour seen as a result of, and a perpetuating factor for, body dysmorphophobic disorder (BDD); although in BDD the focus is not so much the adiposity of stomach or thighs as the size of a nose or chin, texture of complexion or more individual feature. Perceptual distortion in both eating disorders and BDD may be triggered by various psychosocial stimuli including low mood, comparisons with other people's bodies and eating high calorie foods.

Distorted psychological perceptions of appearance can be so intense that they may appear to be downright delusional. The individual's mind may distort actual appearance or may develop overvalued ideas about the way in which other people perceive or judge their physical appearance. Some clinicians have considered the body image distortion in AN to be delusional and have prescribed antipsychotic medications such as olanzapine, not just for their weight gain side effects but to address such 'delusions'.

The present authors have encountered few if any patients whose drive to be exceedingly thin has been based on any delusional belief that they were fat. Patients' attitudes may be formulated as closer to an obsessional fear of fatness, resulting in compulsive 'undoing'

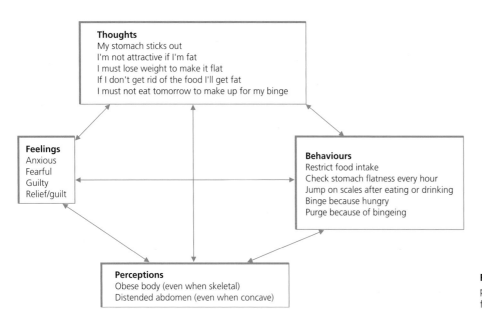

Figure 3.1 The interconnection between perceptions, thoughts, behaviours and feelings.

and 'checking' rituals, and leading to a fear of weight gain that grows with avoidance. In this it is like the OCD fear of contamination, where the patient 'feels' dirty unless they have washed far more than the average person, and engages in 'undoing', checking and avoidance. Antipsychotic medications such as risperidone and olanzapine may allow people with either AN or OCD to tolerate levels of anxiety which would otherwise result in rituals.

Body dissatisfaction

Features of body dissatisfaction include discomfort, complaint and seeking for reassurance about appearance. Increase in body dissatisfaction predicts onset of and increase in dieting and bulimic pathology. Body dissatisfaction has been identified as a motivator to lose weight. Dissatisfaction with a skeletal body might logically be expected to motivate some patients to regain a healthier weight, but sadly in practice the reverse seems more likely. Body dissatisfaction in both AN and BN has been ascribed to both cultural/societal views and personality. Thinness is culturally valued and encouraged by the Western media (especially through magazine exposure) and body dissatisfaction is assisted by the internalization of thin ideals (Tiggemann 2003). The controversy as to whether media images 'cause' eating disorders has been hotly debated, but there is little doubt that they provide a rich culture medium for pre-existing body image dissatisfaction.

'Body checking' behaviours

Body dissatisfaction can lead to either avoidance of self-images or an obsessive search for reassurance—or indeed some combination of these. Only the youngest, most naïve patients rely on reassurance from others, and most resort to secretive forms of self-reassurance, which turn into a vigilant search for imperfection. Behaviours include excessive grooming, looking in the mirror at perceived defects (or for narcissistic gratification at low weight) and frequent weighing. Body dissatisfaction or vigilance may be maintained by checking behaviours, such as assessing fat by pinching and measuring specific areas, and using certain garments and clothes sizes as reference points. Checking and comparing with others and with media figures is frequent. In recent years, self-photography, using webcams and mobile phone cameras has become common.

In contrast, checking may be avoided altogether out of self-consciousness or fear of attention regarding appearance. New information with which to challenge negative assumptions is thus unavailable. The perceived problem area may be hidden with large clothes or a posture adopted that covers it up. Seeing one's reflection in mirrors or windows may be avoided and activities such as swimming which demand body-revealing costumes become impossible. In the extreme sufferers become housebound and socially isolated for fear of exposing their bodily appearance. Engagement in either avoidance or checking behaviours can vary depending on such factors as interpersonal interactions, mood, weight and eating changes.

Such preoccupation with one's appearance is both distressing and time consuming. Sadly, it is on a spectrum of behaviours which are cultural norms for many young women. It is unlikely

however that obsessive grooming is a purely modern phenomenon, since the appearance of young people and especially young women has always served as a signal of health and potential fertility to prospective mates.

Body image and self-esteem

In modern Western society a slim body image is closely linked to self-esteem. Dieting and exercise programmes alongside beauty treatments and surgery are seen as a way of increasing self-esteem even in the healthy population, but far more so for eating disorder subjects. Meanwhile, avoidance of social situations where a person's body is on display, may lead to isolation, a secondary decrease in self-esteem and an increase in depressive symptomatology. However, one interesting finding is that cognitive behavioural interventions for self-esteem can improve a negative body image without necessarily targeting specific body image concerns (Lavallee & Cash 1997) and general self-esteem and empowerment programmes in schools and colleges are more likely to diminish incidence of eating disorders than programmes specifically raising awareness of eating disorders (Piran *et al.* 1999).

Treatments to improve body image

Various treatment approaches and exercises used to normalize body image disturbance are represented in Table 3.2. A recent review of empirically evaluated treatments by Farrell *et al.* (2006) concluded that cognitive behavioural therapy (CBT) is the most empirically supported of these. However, it is extraordinarily difficult to make comparisons and to dissect out answers to some important questions.

Much of the existing scant evidence base has been gathered using subjects who have no diagnosable eating disorder and most subjects have been young and female. It seems unlikely that a single

Table 3.2 Treatments for disorders of body image. (From Cash & Pruzinsky 2004, p. 470)

Mental representation approaches	Sensory techniques
Imagery	Music therapy
Client generated imagery (non directed)	Dance/movement therapy
Guided body image techniques	Art therapy
Hypnosis	Massage and self-touch
Journal writing	
Metaphor and poetry therapy	
Affirmations	
Somatic techniques	Integrated approaches
Breathing exercises	Psychodrama
Relaxation exercises	Bioenergetics
Body awareness exercises	Body talk
Massage therapy	Family sculpting
Rolfing	Focusing (Eugene Gendlin)
Alexander technique	Gestalt therapy
Feldenkrais methods	Somatic experiencing (Peter Levine)
	Synergy (Ilana Rubenfeld)

approach to body image acceptance can be recommended for all, whether or not they have suffered from an eating disorder currently or in the past. We do not yet know which aspects of the body image construct should be prioritized in different cases.

A great range of measures, ranging from subjective estimates of 'feelings of fatness' to complex 'EGON apparatus', has been used in assessing body image change, with little work on validity of these. For instance, mirror exposure or video feedback may result in more accurate size estimation, but there are conflicting reports of how useful this may be in terms of acceptance of an 'imperfect' appearance.

It is important to consider, given recognition of 'body checking' as a perpetuating factor, that inappropriate attention to body image may increase rather than decrease the chances of weight-losing disorders. In addition, such work might inadvertently retraumatize people who have been abused, although non-verbal dance and movement, music and art therapies have been specifically tailored to be used with traumatized patients.

Treatment setting

Referrals for body image interventions are best made to specialist eating disorders clinics, though psychologists, physiotherapists, art, dance and movement therapists, feminist therapists and even family therapists have all staked claims to delivery of such treatments, and CBT (currently the best-evidenced treatment) may be available from clinicians of virtually any discipline in all settings. Timing of body image work may affect outcome in AN. Even high-functioning intellectual performance does not guarantee deeper reflective capacity in a starved brain. Equally importantly, a low weight patient may feel proud of her emaciated body, so that the sort of 'exposure and response prevention' therapy that involves tolerating the discomfort

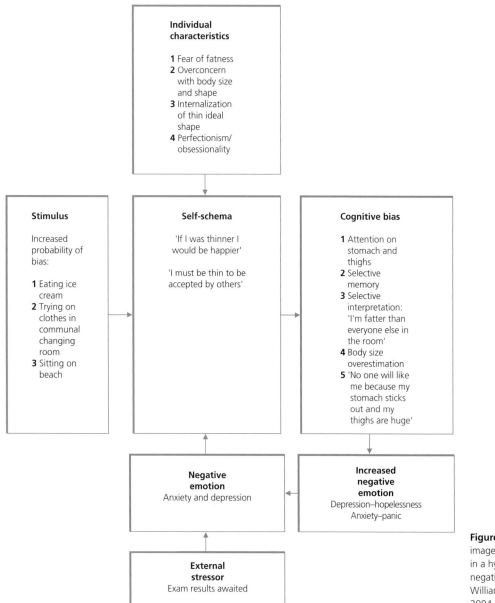

Figure 3.2 Cognitive model of body image as it may apply to eating disorders in a hypothetical individual, highlighting the negative feedback loop. (Adapted from Williamson *et al.* in Cash and Pruzinsky 2004, p. 48)

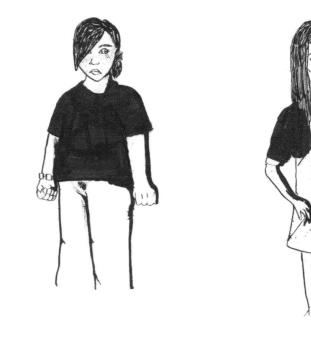

Figure 3.3 Katie, who is emaciated as a result of anorexia nervosa has drawn her own self-portrait (a) and a portrait of her friend (b). Katie's perception of her own appearance is closely linked to her associated distress—the figure is weeping because it 'feels fat'. It is interesting that Katie has drawn her friend as apparently of normal weight—the friend too has low weight anorexia and appears to observers to be much thinner than this.

(a)

(b)

of an unwanted body image is not possible. It may be more effective when at least some weight restoration has been achieved, perhaps as a 'predischarge' intervention.

There are pros and cons to group treatments, given that social avoidance may be involved. Multidiagnostic groups including both bulimic and anorexic patients may experience particularly destructive dynamics. Group packages have several advantages: economic, psycho-education, exposure and response prevention. Groups also provide the opportunity for behavioural experiments in a protected interpersonal milieu. The need, however, to select, screen and prepare patients for group work militates against apparent economic benefits. Individual self-help psycho-educational packages are cheap and private; however, they require motivation for successful outcome.

Cognitive behavioural techniques for body image disturbance in eating disorders

Cognitive behavioural therapy is widely acknowledged as the leading treatment for BN and binge eating disorder (NICE 2004). Cash's (1997) CBT intervention for body shape concern in the USA has been successful for subjects experiencing body image distress, though not always in the presence of a diagnosable eating disorder. A cognitive model of body image and eating disorders represents the feedback loop of negative emotion triggering body image self-schemas, which in turn induce negative emotion (Figures 3.2–3.4).

Fairburn *et al.*'s (2003) 'transdiagnostic' CBT model for eating disorders is designed to include those with comorbid conditions such as substance abuse as well as those who fall into the AN weight range. It adds new modules on top of the basic CBT model. One striking addition is that of body checking and avoidance.

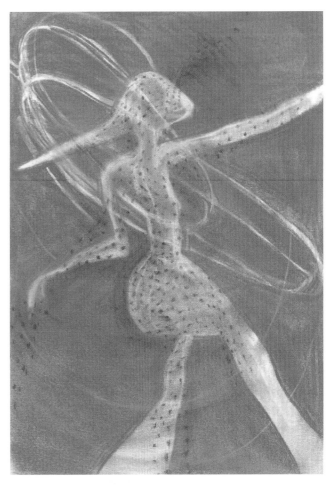

Figure 3.4 Betsy says she feels energized by being so thin and has provided a red background because 'red represents the anorexic community to which I am proud to belong'.

There is a dearth of treatment relating specifically to body image within the eating disorder self-help packages. The main focus of these packages (which will be discussed further in Chapter 9) is bingeing and purging. On the other hand Cash's (1997) self-help *Body Image Workbook* is not specifically aimed at people with formal eating disorders.

Conclusion and recommendations

Body image is a central, schema-based key to all eating disorders and predicts the stability of recovery. Body image concerns and related behaviours such as checking and avoidance are rarely addressed in current therapy packages. Cognitive behavioural therapy, in the context of specific eating disorders treatment, offers the best evidence-based treatment so far.

Further reading

Bruch H. Perceptual and conceptual disturbances in anorexia nervosa. *Psychosomatic Medicine* 1962; **24**: 187–194.

Cash TF. *The Body Image Workbook: An Eight-step Program for Learning to Like Your Looks.* Harbinger, Oakland, CA, 1997.

Cash TF & Pruzinsky T. *Body Image: A Handbook of Theory, Research and Clinical Practice.* Guilford, New York, 2004.

Collins JK, Beumont PJV, Touyz S *et al.* Variability in body shape perception in anorexic, bulimic, obese, and control subjects. *International Journal of Eating Disorders* 1987; **6**: 633–638.

Fairburn CG, Cooper Z & Shafran R. Cognitive behaviour therapy for eating disorders: a 'transdiagnostic' theory and treatment. *Behaviour Research and Therapy* 2003; **41**: 509–528.

Farrell C, Shafran R & Lee M. Empirically evaluated treatments for body image disturbance: a review. *European Eating Disorders Review* 2006; **14**: 289–300.

Farrell C, Shafran R, Lee M & Fairburn CG. Testing a brief cognitive-behavioural intervention to improve extreme shape concern: a case series. *Behavioural and Cognitive Psychotherapy* 2005; **33**(2): 189–200.

Marcus MD, Smith D, Santelli R & Kaye W. Characterization of eating disordered behaviour in obese binge eaters. *International Journal of Eating Disorders* 1992; **1**: 249–255.

NICE. *Eating Disorders: Core Interventions in the Treatment and Management of Anorexia Nervosa, Bulimia Nervosa and Related Eating Disorders.* NICE Clinical Guideline No 9. National Institute for Clinical Excellence, London, 2004: http://www.nice.org.uk

Shafran R & Robinson P. Thought-shape fusion in eating disorders. *British Journal of Clinical Psychology* 2004; **43**: 399–408.

Tiggemann M. Media exposure, body dissatisfaction and disordered eating: television and magazines are not the same! *International Journal of Eating Disorders* 2003; **11**: 418–430.

CHAPTER 4

Compulsive Exercise and Overactivity in Eating Disorders

Jane Morris

OVERVIEW

- Exercise and overactivity may be one route into so-called 'eating disorders', and often coexist with dietary restriction, purging and other weight-losing behaviours.

- Male sufferers and elite athletes may seek a lean, muscular body image in preference to mere thinness and will use exercise (and perhaps drugs of abuse) rather than diet alone to achieve this.

- Overexercise causes endorphin release and may result in a picture which resembles both addictive and obsessive-compulsive psychopathology.

- Starved animals—including humans—may become paradoxically hyperactive, agitated and aggressive. This, together with the drive to lose weight and burn calories, results in bizarre compulsive overactivity such as the inability to sit still or even sit down at all.

- Weight-recovered patients who continue to overexercise have a worse prognosis.

- Programmes that reintroduce healthy ways to exercise are only recently becoming available.

Exercise as a component of 'eating' disorders (Figure 4.1 and Boxes 4.1 & 4.2)

In modern Western cultures anorexia and normal weight bulimia nervosa are usually linked to aesthetic overvaluation of thinness. The term 'eating disorders' is misleading though: self-starvation is only one way to make bodies leaner. Methods of attempted weight reduction, including vomiting, purging using laxatives or diuretics, 'rumination' (chewing and spitting out food), abuse of slimming pills, thyroxine, stimulants, underuse of insulin, tolerating cold and extreme levels of physical activity. Excessive running was described as an analogue of anorexia by Yates *et al.* in 1983.

Compulsive activity may not resemble normal 'exercise'. Its hallmarks are oddness and secrecy. Sufferers undertake repeated sit-ups and pushups in locked bathrooms, take more exercise or dance classes than anyone realises, do incessant housework, walk dogs for

miles, even set alarms to exercise whilst others are sleeping. This is compounded by standing rather than sitting, leg twitching and fidgeting when obliged to sit or lie down, making excuses to 'go to the bathroom', fetching one item at a time, 'forgetting' things, and running up and down stairs.

Which patients are particularly likely to experience compulsive exercise and overactivity?

Compulsive exercise is not an invariable part of anorexia nervosa (some develop chronic fatigue) but may be increasing in all eating disordered patients. Glossy magazines now feature more articles on exercise as well as diet. Not everyone can tolerate starvation—exercise offers an alternative. Some volunteers in the Minnesota semi-starvation study (Keys *et al.* 1950) exercised to qualify for an extra calorie allowance. The 'buzz' of exercise may offer a socially sanctioned alternative to drug use and relieve the discomfort of pure starvation.

Male sufferers often value a lean but muscular shape (Whitehead's [1994] 'machismo nervosa') requiring exercise as well as diet. In men, weight and shape preoccupation plus an obsessive-compulsive personality are the strongest predictors of compulsion to exercise (Davis 1993). For women too there is now a fashion for a muscular as well as slim body, exploited by commercial gym and exercise concerns.

There may sometimes be a iatrogenic component. If not already part of the picture, overexercise may appear—like purging—as a response to enforced refeeding. Many treatment programmes even prescribe exercise as a privilege earned by weight gain—risking the exchange of one form of obsessive body control for another.

Eating disorders in elite athletes (Box 4.3)

It is still unknown whether sport and dance 'cause' eating disorders, or attract those who are predisposed to develop them anyway. Overexercise and dieting may be alternative routes to obsessive body control. All attract perfectionist body-conscious strivers, and then amplify these traits. Just as dieters may espouse the external constraints of formal veganism or claim 'allergies' to reinforce their

ABC of Eating Disorders. Edited by J. Morris. © 2008 Blackwell Publishing, ISBN: 978-0-7279-1843-7.

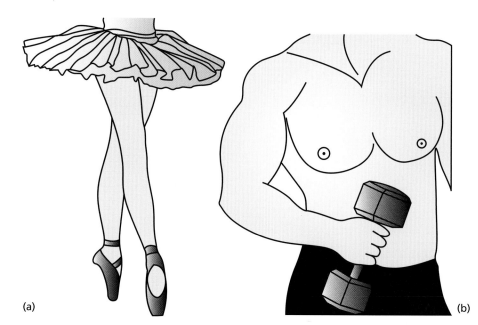

Figure 4.1 Ballerinas face the challenge of having to exercise strenuously on inadequate nutritional supplies in order to keep the body thin, whilst body builders engage in strenuous exercise specifically to build the desired bulky appearance.

(a)

(b)

Box 4.1 **Case vignette: Andy**

Andy played for his school rugby team from first year onwards. Around the time of public exams all but the keenest dropped out, and Andy found himself up against older boys in the first and second teams. The frequency of training was stepped up, with lunchtime gym sessions, and the new coach issued 'healthy diet' sheets as well.

Andy began to lose weight, his performance deteriorated and he had to drop out of the squad with a knee injury. He became low and depressed but continued to go to the gym by himself—he said he felt too guilty to eat unless he had completed a punishing workout. It was only at this stage that he began to develop body image concerns, measuring the circumference of his arms and thighs and drinking special protein-rich concoctions that he ordered from the internet.

Box 4.2 **Hallmarks of healthy exercise**

- Quality rather than just quantity of activity is what counts—if exercise is enjoyable, rather than a desperate duty, it is more likely to be healthy.
- Someone who is healthy can cancel a session of exercise for the sake of injury or social events—healthy exercise does not interfere with other aspects of life.
- Anyone who gets terribly distressed or angry when their exercise is cancelled has an unhealthy attitude towards exercise and needs help.
- Activities undertaken mainly to burn off calories are not healthy.
- 'Odd' activity is unhealthy—e.g. carrying a pile of clothes upstairs one item at a time, refusing lifts in order to walk extra miles, insisting on doing all the family housework, walking to school when classmates take the bus, refusing to sit down when no-one else is standing, constant 'fidgeting'.
- Secret activity is unhealthy activity.
- Beware of counting while exercising.
- There is no *need* to do formal 'exercise' at all, if there are plenty of chances to take walks, play with the family, kick the odd ball around, swim maybe once a week, do light housework and limit time spent in front of screens. Activity should not be 'all or nothing'.

---

own willpower, so overexercisers espouse the formal disciplines of coaching and competition. Ambitious coaches, parents and dance teachers then unwittingly collude. Skating and dancing may be particularly fertile soil for anorexia since mirrors in dance studios and the demands of costumes foster the perpetuating habit of 'body checking'. Jockeys, coxes and boxers are obliged to undergo 'weigh-ins' and performance sports dictate a stereotyped appearance, but even where there is no evidence that low weight enhances performance (in running, for instance) the myth persists that the lower the weight, the better, just as the myth persists that 'healthy' food must be low-calorie food.

Understanding overexercise: obsessive-compulsive or addictive?

Whether or not exercise starts as a considered strategy for burning calories or sculpting muscle, it soon becomes far

more than this. In addition to social approval of exercise and psychological overvaluation of low weight, biological factors amplify the urge to activity.

Famine studies show that the brain's biological response to starvation is to sleep less and become aroused, jittery and even aggressive—perhaps an evolved way to enhance the hunt for food. This is further reinforced by the release of feel-good endorphins from tissue breakdown. Epling *et al.* (1983) showed that overexercise

Box 4.3 **Is it safe to return to serious competitive sport or professional dance after an eating disorder?**

- There is certainly a high risk involved. It is rather like asking whether a former alcoholic can safely enjoy a career as a wine merchant!
- The sooner the return to competitive sport, the higher the risk. It's best to wait 12 months after full weight gain, before taking up serious training again.
- Achieve healthy weight first—and keep minimum weight monitored. Athletic bodies contain a higher proportion of muscle than usual, so normal guidelines on healthy body mass index (BMI) are too low—athletes and dancers need to be heavier than someone with less muscle.
- Girls and women stop menstruating if their weight drops too low—use this as a warning sign. (However, the contraceptive pill causes withdrawal bleeds even at low weight—do not be misled.)
- Start training slowly and patiently. It takes time to rebuild fitness.
- Those who are unable to take 2 days off from physical training each week should see this as a warning that the compulsion is returning.
- Athletes should be prepared to take a substantial break from serious competition in the event of injury or illness—including relapse of the eating disorder.
- Returning athletes are well-advised to have at least one other important interest, in case the career in sport/dance does turn out to be more harmful than beneficial—perhaps art or music for instance.
- Coaches and trainers need to know the medical history and agree to prioritize the individual's health.
- Specialist eating disorders professionals who are independent from the athletic organization should regularly monitor not only nutritional and physical needs but also psychological health.

in starved animals is mediated by endogenous opioid peptides. An 'addiction' model suggests that subjects crave such inherently gratifying sensations regardless of harm, and experience 'withdrawal' if prevented from indulging. Habituation—the need for increasing 'doses' to get the same reward—might explain the need to run that extra lap or swim that extra length each day. Addiction research also warns of the risk of reinstatement after periods of abstinence.

In contrast, Davis *et al.* (1990s) believe commitment to exercise is characteristically obsessional rather than addictive. Obsessive-compulsive behaviours are not inherently pleasurable, but the subject experiences guilt and anxiety if the behaviour is not achieved. Exercise to avoid fatness corresponds to the neutralizing or 'undoing' rituals in classic obsessive compulsive disorder, such as hand washing to counter contamination, or checking to prevent catastrophes. This model would predict that increasing avoidance amplifies anxiety and multiplies rituals.

Certainly many families where there is anorexia nervosa show a genetic predisposition to the obsessive-compulsive spectrum of disorders, and Goldfarb and Plante (1984) found that obsessive personality traits predict frequency of exercise. Obsessive-compulsive

rituals, however, are usually said to be 'ego-dystonic', and to be resisted and known to be ridiculous. This clearly does not apply to exercise, although it may be characteristic of the furtive twitching and fidgeting behaviours. Addictive problems, on the other hand, are more prevalent in the families of bulimic patients, so there may be genetically distinct characteristics of exercise patterns in different eating disorders.

How could exercise help or harm?

Physical exercise takes many different forms, meeting a range of different needs and drives, some healthy, some pathological. Just as binge eating is not a cure for anorexia, becoming a 'couch potato' is hardly a healthy substitute for compulsive exercise. The benefits of relearning a balanced approach to exercise might include preventing overweight, counteracting osteoporosis, increasing cardiovascular fitness, and reducing depression and anxiety (Bouchard *et al.* 1990). All these do, however, depend for their effectiveness on adequate renutrition.

At low weight overactivity causes not only further weight loss but also fatigue, amenorrhoea, infertility, osteoporosis, heat stroke, dehydration, collapse, injury (fractures, head injuries, soft tissue injuries) and overuse damage (arthritis, deformity). Bones are already brittle as a result of starvation (Figure 4.2), and when vertebrae in particular are damaged the result can be permanent kyphosis. Muscle breakdown always results from exercise, but the body of a well-nourished person rebuilds and enhances the muscle. In starvation this cannot happen. Heart muscle suffers breakdown too, and the heart shrinks and slows down in response to the limited energy available. Many deaths from anorexia are a result of cardiac problems. Ninety per cent of eating disorders mortality occurs in winter months, and overexercise may contribute significantly to this. Those who focus on getting their exercise to the exclusion of other concerns are more likely to have accidents or injuries, unable to build a healthy immune system and vulnerable to hypothermia as well as infections.

Another overlooked risk is the associated abuse of drugs. Anabolic steroids amplify mood swings and aggression, whilst painkillers permit continuing tissue destruction and may damage the liver and gastrointestinal tract.

Psychologically, exercise which becomes compulsive loses its pleasurable, playful aspect, and prevents concentration on education or interpersonal activities—some people cannot even sit down in school! Overcompetitive exercise may lead to circumscribed conditional measures of self-esteem and self-punishing attitudes. Social activities are sacrificed as other people are seen as mere obstacles to the relentless exercise schedule.

Could exercise promote recovery? (Box 4.4)

Despite theoretical concerns, some studies suggest that prescribed exercise programmes may be helpful in engaging low weight patients in treatment. Many respected treatment centres offer exercise opportunities with a focus on quality rather than quantity of exercise—yoga and tai chi, for instance. The University of British Columbia (Thien *et al.* 2000) conducted a randomized study of

Referring Physician: **MORRIS**

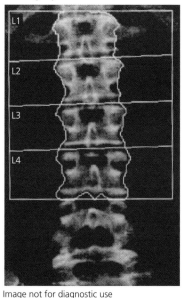

Image not for diagnostic use
116×129

Scan Information:
Scan Date: 25 August 2006
Scan Type: a Lumbar Spine
Analysis: 25 August 2006 11:03 Version 11.2
    Lumbar Spine
Operator: CM
Model: QDR 4500A (S/N 45666)
Comment:

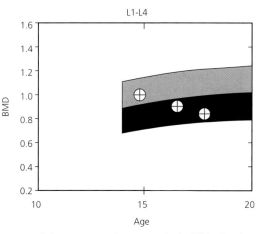

L1-L4

Reference curve and scores matched to White Female
Source: Hologic

DXA Results Summary:

Scan Date	Age	BMD (g/cm²)	T - Score	BMD Change vs Baseline	vs Previous
25.08.2006	17	0.840	−1.9	−15.7%*	−6.7%*
19.05.2005	16	0.901	−1.3	−9.6%*	−9.6%*
19.08.2003	14	0.997	−0.5		

Total BMD CV 1.0%
* Denotes significant change at the 95% confidence level.

Figure 4.2 This young girl maintained a steady weight in the normal range but was exercising heavily and menstruating only intermittently. Her bone mineral density has dropped well below average although it is not yet in the 'osteoporotic' range.

graded exercise versus treatment as usual for patients with anorexia nervosa, followed up for 3 months. Surprisingly there was no difference in either rate of weight gain or percentage body fat between the two groups. Less surprisingly, patients preferred the exercise programme.

How can an understanding of overexercise promote recovery and prevent relapse?

Compulsive exercise in eating disorders has been found to correlate with worse prognosis (Penas-Liedo *et al.* 2002)—perhaps because it is rarely adequately addressed. The first essential is a climate of greater awareness of exercise compulsion as a life-damaging problem rather than merely a nuisance interfering with weight gain.

Most attention is paid to the dangers of overactivity when patients present to hospital in extremis, when warmth and rest may be life-saving. Complete bed rest is not proven to be helpful and may exacerbate pressure sores, but patients may need constant observation and gentle restraint alongside repeated explanation and reassurance. Benzodiazepines or olanzapine are probably the safest sedatives for a starved body. Observation in bathrooms may be the only way to ensure that 'resting' patients do not engage in frenetic exercise under the pretence of using the toilet or taking a shower. Skilled nurses combine firmness and delicacy to undertake this task with compassion.

During renutrition it is crucial to monitor increased activity without allowing a rigid 'calorie economy' to give the message of exchanging one anorexic behaviour for another. We should teach the ability to rest, relax and recuperate as a highly desirable skill in the arsenal of self-care. It is more effective to positively prescribe normal sedentary activities such as card and board games or crafts, rather than ban unhealthy behaviours. Tai chi and yoga are gentle, non-competitive activities fostering balance, grace and relaxation. Training in alternative stress-management skills may help too. Cognitive techniques can help patients identify and then conduct experiments to test out anorexic beliefs such as 'if I don't do 50 press-ups each night I will gain 10 kg in a week'. Antidepressant medication is notoriously ineffectual in low weight patients but a trial of selective serotonin reuptake inhibitors (SSRIs) in higher, antiobsessive doses may be warranted, especially if obsessive compulsive disorder predates the eating disorder.

Weltzin *et al.* (1991) made the intriguing observation that recovered 'restricting' anorexia sufferers have increased calorie requirements compared with controls and former bulimic-subtype patients. It is possible that this reflects the use of excessive exercise in 'non-purging' anorexia. Anecdotally, 'recovered' eating disorder patients often still use a great deal of exercise and commonly 'celebrate' recovery with demanding physical challenges such as sponsored marathons.

Box 4.4 **Starting exercise and activity during recovery from eating disorders**

- Tai chi fosters balance, strength, relaxation and calm—and can be done whilst sitting down at first.
- Activities like table football, darts, snooker and pool are opportunities to introduce sport and games in a gentle way, and to learn to be playful rather than ruthlessly competitive.
- Swimming, bowling, 'putting' or crazy golf, croquet, walking and yoga are good to move on to. These often involve going outdoors, so need to be planned more carefully, with appropriate clothing.
- Exercise needs to be supervised so that someone can point out problems such as 'trying too hard'. Schools, clubs and group leaders all need to help—it is asking far too much to expect the eating disorder sufferer to fight the compulsion alone at this stage.
- Even when someone seems recovered, it is a good safeguard to chose social rather than solitary exercise—rambler groups rather than solitary running, yoga classes rather than the gym.
- Make sure exercise sessions are no longer than 30 minutes at a time, and no more than 3 days a week at first. The ability to tolerate 'rest days' is crucial.
- Be aware of 'incidental' exercise—walking to school or work, shopping, housework, etc. There is little point taking great care with swimming sessions if the person walks miles to and from the pool on a dark cold night with wet hair and light clothing!
- Be prepared for the early return to exercise to feel very frustrating at first—remind the person that new values are in place—be suspicious of the 'high' or the 'burn', exercising in deadly earnest, or if there is upset when not winning or beating a personal best.
- Deliberately practise both physical and mental relaxation as well as exercise—consider meditation, mindfulness, flotation, gentle massage (if tolerated).
- As people gain weight it is tempting to do special exercises to 'sculpt' the body—for instance situps to trim stomach muscles. This risks strains or even hernias. All-over activity is best, trusting the body's wisdom to redistribute energy in healthy proportions over time.
- Notice what happens to weight. If it does not continue to move steadily towards the healthiest body mass index (BMI), then activity and eating are out of balance.
- Notice what happens to social life—those who spend more time relating to other people (**not** just exercising beside them, or competing with them!) are genuinely recovering.

Even return to otherwise healthy levels of physical exercise may be physically dangerous early in weight recovery. Bone building takes many months, so starvation-induced osteopaenia persists for several years after recovery, with associated fracture risk. Contact sports, gymnastics, skiing, skating and horse riding should wait until bone scans show improved density.

Further reading

Bouchard C, Shephard RJ, Stephens T *et al.*, eds. *Exercise, Fitness and Health.* Human Kinetics, Champaign, Illinois, 1990.

Davis C, Kennedy SH, Ravelski E & Dionne M. The role of physical activity in the development and maintenance of eating disorders. *Psychological Medicine* 1994; **24**: 957–967.

Epling WF, Pierce WD & Stefan L. A theory of activity-based anorexia. *International Journal of Eating Disorders* 1983; **3**(1): 27–43.

Goldfarb LA & Plante TG. Fear of fat in runners: an examination of the connection between anorexia nervosa and distance running. *Psychological Review* 1984; **55**: 296.

Keys A, Brozek J, Henschel A, Mickelson O & Taylor HL. *The Biology of Human Starvation.* University of Minnesota, Minneapolis, 1950.

Penas-Liedo E, Vaz Leal FJ & Waller G. Excessive exercise in anorexia nervosa and bulimia nervosa: relation to eating characteristics and general psychopathology. *International Journal of Eating Disorders* 2002; **31**: 370–75.

Thien V, Thomas A, Markin L *et al.* Pilot study of a graded exercise program for the treatment of anorexia nervosa. *International Journal of Eating Disorders* 2000; **28**(1): 101–106.

Weltzin TE, Fernstrom MH, Hansen D *et al.* Abnormal caloric requirements for weight maintenance in patients with anorexia and bulimia nervosa. *American Journal of Psychiatry* 1991; **148**: 1675–1682.

Whitehead L. Machismo nervosa: a new type of eating disorder in men. *International Cognitive Therapy Newsletter* 1994; **8**(2): 3.

Yates A. *Compulsive Exercise and the Eating Disorders: Towards an Integrated Theory of Activity.* Brunner/Mazel, New York, 1991.

CHAPTER 5

Medical and Psychological Consequences of Eating Disorders

Geoffrey Wolff and Janet Treasure

OVERVIEW

- Eating disorders carry a high morbidity and mortality.
- Patients with eating disorders require a thorough assessment of both medical and psychiatric risk.
- Most of the medical and psychological sequelae of eating disorders resolve with treatment of the eating disorder.
- In some cases it may be appropriate for general practitioners and psychiatrists managing patients with eating disorders to involve a physician with expertise with managing the physical consequences of eating disorders.

Introduction

Eating disorders are associated with high levels of both physical and psychological morbidity.

Indeed, patients often initially present to their general practitioner with gynaecological (amenorrhoea, irregular periods), gastrointestinal (constipation, diarrhoea [secondary to laxative abuse]) and psychological (depression, anxiety) symptoms (Ogg *et al.* 1997) (Figure 5.1).

The physical morbidity can affect all body systems (Rome & Ammerman 2003) (Figure 5.2 and Boxes 5.1 & 5.2). Whilst the physical morbidity is essentially mainly secondary to the eating disorder, the relationship with psychological morbidity is more complex. Psychological morbidity and also so-called 'comorbidity' may be integral to the disorder as well as being at the same time both cause and consequence of the disorder. The psychological consequences discussed in this chapter therefore must be seen in this context.

Many of the physical and psychological consequences result from starvation as illustrated by the starvation study in healthy volunteers by Ancel Keys (Keys *et al.* 1950) (Box 5.3).

Eating disorders in general are also associated with marked impairment of quality of life through: lack of energy, emotional distress, social isolation and sleep disturbance (Keilen *et al.* 1994).

Anorexia nervosa in particular is also associated with high levels of chronic disability from, for example, reduced mobility

ABC of Eating Disorders. Edited by J. Morris. © 2008 Blackwell Publishing, ISBN: 978-0-7279-1843-7.

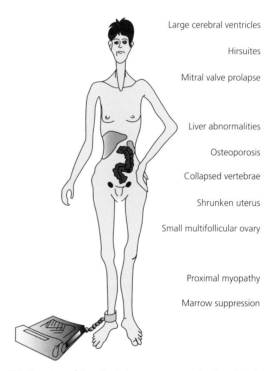

Large cerebral ventricles

Hirsuites

Mitral valve prolapse

Liver abnormalities

Osteoporosis

Collapsed vertebrae

Shrunken uterus

Small multifollicular ovary

Proximal myopathy

Marrow suppression

Figure 5.1 Overview of the physical consequences of eating disorders.

and pain (Box 5.4). The mortality from anorexia nervosa is 10 times that of general population and twice that of other psychiatric inpatients (Sullivan 1995; Nielsen *et al.* 1998; Herzog *et al.* 2000). The main causes of death are infections, cardiovascular collapse and suicide. There are high levels of psychiatric comorbidity including depression, obsessive compulsive disorder and social phobia, and suicide rates are higher than for any psychiatric disorder and are 60 times that of general population (Herzog *et al.* 2000). Patients with anorexia nervosa tend to have anxious, obsessional and avoidant personality traits. They also complain that their illness causes them to feel out of control, taken over, preoccupied with thoughts about food, and that it damages their personal relationships.

Bulimia nervosa is also associated with high levels of psychiatric comorbidity including depression and substance abuse (Box 5.5). Bulimia nervosa sufferers tend to have borderline and impulsive

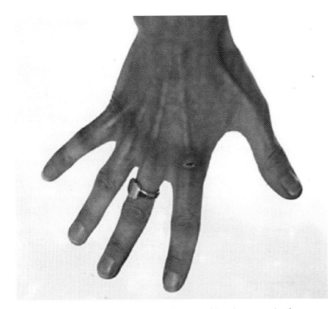

Figure 5.2 Russell's sign. (Callous on dorsum of hand as a result of inducing vomiting.)

Box 5.1 **Presentation of eating disorders in general practice**

Gynaecological complaints
- Amenorrhea
- Irregular periods

Gastrointestinal complaints
- Constipation
- Diarrhoea

Psychological complaints
- Depression
- Anxiety

Box 5.2 **External surfaces**

- Dry flaky skin with no collagen
- Lanugo hair
- Poor peripheral circulation, Raynauds, perniosis
- Petechial rash from thrombocytopenia, scurvy
- Brittle nails
- Carotenaemia
- Russell's sign—callous on metacarpophalangeal joint (see Figure 5.2)
- Facial purpura (increased intrathoracic pressure with vomiting)
- Conjunctival haemorrhage (increased intrathoracic pressure)

Box 5.3 **The Minnesota data (Keys *et al.* 1950)**

- Apathy and lethargy
- Ritualistic eating habits—obsessive
- Preoccupation with food—narrowed interests
- Craving and hunger
- Emotional blunting
- Irritability and nervousness
- Low mood
- Poor sleep
- ↓ Libido
- Body image distortion
- Poor concentration
- ↓ Capacity for work
- IQ normal, but slow
- ↓ Personality
- ↓ Sociability/social phobia

Box 5.4 **Morbidity and mortality in anorexia nervosa**

- Functional gastrointestinal disorders
- Osteoporosis
- Infertility
- Depression
- Death due to:
  infections
  cardiovascular collapse
  suicide

Box 5.5 **Morbidity and mortality in bulimia nervosa**

- Dental erosion
- Depression
- Death due to:
  suicide
  cardiac arrhythmias

Box 5.6 **Risk areas in eating disorders**

- Fasting, starvation and weight loss
- Compensatory strategies:
  vomiting
  laxative abuse
- Bingeing
- Refeeding

---

personality traits. Medical comorbidity is less than that for anorexia nervosa. Patients with bulimia nervosa complain that their illness causes them to feel shame or low self-esteem and leads to obsessive thoughts about weight and shape.

Atypical eating disorders (or eating disorders not otherwise specified) are even more common than both anorexia nervosa and bulimia nervosa combined. Levels of distress and disability are comparable to those seen in anorexia nervosa and bulimia nervosa.

Different eating disorders share common features and symptom patterns change over time. In considering medical and psychological consequences, therefore, we will, as far as possible, consider the consequences of specific features and behaviours associated with eating disorders rather than diagnostic categories (Box 5.6). These include:
- fasting and starvation plus weight loss;
- weight-control strategies (vomiting and laxative abuse);
- bingeing.

Furthermore, in low weight patients weight restoration or refeeding carries its own complications and these are also discussed.

One caveat, however, is that causal relationships may be complex with some complications such as electrolyte disturbances being secondary to a combination of factors.

Medical and psychological consequences of starvation and weight loss

Endocrine system

Hypothalamic–pituitary–gonadal (HPG) axis—The HPG axis regresses to that of a prepubertal child. The pituitary does not secrete follicle-stimulating hormone (FSH) and luteinizing hormone (LH) and the ovaries decrease in size. The ovarian follicles remain small and do not produce oestrogens or progesterone.

The hypothalamic–pituitary–thyroid (HPT) axis—Hypothyroidism may occur with reduced T3 and T4 with normal TSH levels. (Reverse T3 can be increased.)

The hypothalamic–pituitary–adrenal (HPA) axis—The HPA axis is overactive, probably driven by excess corticotropin-releasing factor (CRF), with high levels of cortisol which are not constrained by any feedback.

Growth hormone—This is increased in about 50% of patients with anorexia nervosa.

Reproductive function

Amenorrhoea tends to occur below a body mass index (BMI) of 17.5. Fertility is therefore reduced in women with anorexia nervosa. Reduced fertility rates persist over a long time frame, in part due to suboptimal physical recovery. Indeed, in a follow up of 12.5 years in Denmark the fertility rate was a third of that expected.

Women with anorexia nervosa also have significantly more miscarriages and caesarean deliveries, and the perinatal mortality rate is around sixfold higher than the normal population.

The offspring of women with anorexia nervosa are significantly more likely to be born prematurely and are of lower birth weight than the offspring of controls.

Furthermore, women with anorexia nervosa may also have difficulties in feeding their children, who may become malnourished and stunted in growth.

Skeletal system

Osteoporosis is one of the most severe complications of anorexia nervosa and treatment is uncertain. A diet with adequate amounts of calcium and vitamin D is recommended. The majority of people with anorexia nervosa consume low-fat diets and are likely to be deficient in both.

Osteoporosis and pathological fractures are the commonest causes of pain and disability in anorexia nervosa. The annual incidence of non-spine fractures of 0.05 per person per year in anorexia nervosa is seven-fold higher than the rate reported from a community sample of women aged 15–34 years. Risk factors for this

complication are a long duration and increased severity of illness. In children and adolescents there may be growth retardation and short stature.

Cardiovascular system

The heart becomes smaller and less powerful because muscle is lost. Blood pressure and heart rate is lowered. This can lead to faints. There is poor circulation in the periphery and this leads to cold blue hands, feet and nose. At its extreme, this results in chilblains and even gangrene, particularly in children.

Sudden death has been known to occur in anorexia nervosa and may result from arrhythmias. The risk is higher where there is QT prolongation which is common in anorexia nervosa due to low weight, especially where there is also hypokalaemia which results from vomiting, laxative and diuretic abuse. Indeed, hypotension, bradycardia and QT prolongation may also occur in bulimia nervosa.

Haematology/immune system

All components of the bone marrow are diminished but the order in which this is discernible in the peripheral blood is white cells, red cells and finally platelets. The level of marrow dysfunction relates to the total body fat mass. The immune system is compromised, with a decrease in CD8 T cells. Indeed around one third of deaths due to anorexia nervosa are due to infections such as bronchial pneumonia and sepsis (Zipfel *et al.* 2000).

Gastrointestinal tract

The vast majority of patients with eating disorders have functional gastrointestinal disorders such as irritable bowel syndrome, functional abdominal bloating and functional constipation (Boyd *et al.* 2005). The symptoms improve markedly with weight restoration but residual gastrointestinal problems such as irritable bowel syndrome remain common after recovery from anorexia nervosa (Waldholtz & Andersen 1990). Functional abnormalities such as delayed gastric emptying and generalized poor motility are related to the degree of undernutrition. Anatomical abnormalities as a result of the trauma of vomiting and overeating or loss of mesenteric fat occur. Structural abnormalities such as ulcers are common. It is important not to overlook the effects of sorbitol present in sugar-free gums and sweets, which can cause abdominal distension, cramps, and diarrhoea. Fatty liver may occur.

Central nervous system

Brain substance decreases in anorexia nervosa and the ventricular spaces and the sulci increase in size. To a degree these structural abnormalities, such as loss of gray matter, persist despite weight recovery for over a year, which suggests that there may be a degree of irreversible damage even in adolescents with a short history. The cause of the cerebral atrophy is uncertain. It may be a general effect of starvation or may result from the high level of cortisol, which is present in anorexia nervosa and which is known to be toxic to dendrites.

Functional cognitive impairment is seen with deficits in memory tasks, flexibility and inhibitory tasks persisting despite weight recovery. Women with eating disorders also have weak central coherence, a trait in which there is a bias to detail at the expense of contextual integration (a trait shared with autistic spectrum disorders). Women who have recovered from anorexia nervosa have average IQ scores.

Muscular system

Individuals with severe anorexia nervosa have poor muscle strength and a decrease in stamina. Proximal myopathy is a useful marker of severe physiological compromise. It can be elicited by asking the patient to stand from a crouched position. This symptom indicates the need for urgent nutritional rehabilitation and inpatient treatment.

Neurological system

Peripheral neuropathy may occur occasionally where weight loss is severe.

Renal system

Renal stones and acute renal failure may result from dehydration.

Skin and hair changes

The skin is dry and fine, downy, lanugo hair develops. There is often loss of head hair and what is left appears thin and lifeless.

Metabolic system

Metabolic rate decreases with weight loss and there may be impaired temperature regulation with hypothermia. Hypoglycaemia is common. Hypercholesterolaemia occurs in around 50% of patients with anorexia nervosa.

Electrolyte disturbance

Calcium—Hypocalcaemia is secondary to chronic malnutrition (and also metabolic alkalosis) and may result in tetany and electrocardiogram (ECG) changes as well as osteopaenia or osteoporosis.

Phosphate—Starvation may lead to the depletion of phosphate, which is imperative in cardiac muscle functioning. The requirements for phosphate will increase through refeeding and the demands placed on the heart are also increased. Care must be taken when nutritional therapy is instituted to avoid refeeding syndrome (one of the key components of which is depletion of phosphate).

Iron—Iron deficiency may lead to anaemia.

Zinc—Zinc deficiency may occur rarely and lead to fatigue and mood disturbance.

Vitamins

Vitamin deficiency is unusual in eating disorders. Protection from this deficiency usually comes as a result of low-fat diets usually including a large amount of water-soluble vitamins in the form of fruit and vegetables. In anorexia nervosa, metabolic activity is at a minimal level; an example is that the thiamine required for carbohydrate metabolism is required at much lower levels than people on a balanced diet. A general vitamin and mineral supplements is recommended to supplement nutritional rehabilitation.

Psychological consequences

When considering the psychological (including social and behavioural) features seen in fasting and starvation in eating disorders it is not possible to tease out fully how much is cause and how much consequence. However, the famous Minnesota starvation study confirmed that most of the following psychological features seen in eating disorders are also consequences of fasting and starvation in normal (male) volunteers.

There is a dramatic increase in food preoccupation and poor concentration on their usual activities due to being plagued by incessant thoughts of food and eating. Obsessive behaviour increases around both food-related and other issues. Social withdrawal and isolation increase with growing feelings of social inadequacy.

Even eating small amounts may lead to feeling greedy especially where bloating is experienced or dietary rules are broken. There is an increase in emotional distress with anxiety, depression, mood swings, anger, shame, guilt and feelings of disgust. Episodes of binge eating increase due to both starvation and emotional distress and are followed by self-reproach. Sufferers may feel hopeless and suicidal. Indeed, suicide rates are extremely high in anorexia nervosa (see above).

Complications of weight control strategies: vomiting, laxative and diuretic abuse

Electrolyte disturbance

Hypokalaemia—Hypokalaemia associated with eating disorders is secondary to vomiting as well as laxative and diuretic abuse. It is therefore common in patients with anorexia nervosa of the binge-purge type and lower weight bulimia nervosa (who vomit and/or abuse laxatives)—but rare in pure restricting anorexia nervosa even at very low weight (Greenfeld *et al.* 1995). Indeed in bulimia nervosa the incidence is around 7% compared to 1% in normal controls—rising to over 40% in bulimics who purge at least twice daily (Wolfe *et al.* 2001). Hypokalaemia may result in muscle weakness, cardiac arrhythmias, decreased gut motility and renal tubular dysfunction.

Hyponatraemia—This may result from hypotonic dehydration caused by chronic purging. It may also result from excess water intake. It may result in lethargy and weakness as well as seizures, coma and death.

Fluid balance/acid–base balance—Vomiting may lead to dehydration which can lead to circulatory failure and prerenal failure. Vomiting may also cause metabolic alkalosis which may lead to hypocalcaemia (see above). Abuse of laxatives can produce a metabolic acidosis.

Gastrointestinal

Dental changes—The commonest stigma of persistent vomiting is erosion of dental enamel, in particular from the inner surfaces of

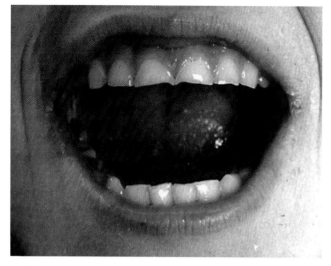

Figure 5.3 Dental erosion.

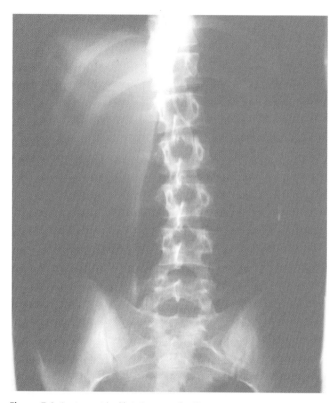

Figure 5.4 Acute gastric dilatation on refeeding.

the front teeth (Figure 5.3). Eventually dentine is exposed and the teeth become oversensitive to temperature and cavities develop. Complications such as abnormal tooth wear are not limited to the group that vomit, however. Other causes of poor dental health are over consumption of acidic foods such as fruit and carbonated drinks, or grinding and loosening of the teeth due to osteoporosis of the jaw.

Salivary glands—A non-inflammatory swelling of the salivary glands is frequently found in the parotids of people with bulimia nervosa (secondary to vomiting). The exact factors underlying salivary gland enlargement in bulimia remains unknown, but it is thought that the increased level of amylase is probably produced by the salivary gland. Raised serum amylase secondary to swollen parotid glands, especially during refeeding and in the presence of abdominal pain may need to be distinguished from that due to pancreatitis which may be a consequence of refeeding.

Gut trauma—Oesophagitis, Mallory–Weiss tears and gastrointestinal bleeding may occur due to vomiting.

Cardiovascular

Arrhythmias may occur secondary to electrolyte disturbance (e.g. hypokalaemia). Hypotension may occur secondary to dehydration.

Kidneys

The misuse of laxatives and vomiting may affect renal function through hypokalaemia and volume depletion. The breakdown of renal function may arise from a reduced glomerular filtration rate (GFR) or renal (kidney) tubular damage (RTD). The term 'renal insufficiency' is used to refer to the mild effect of this condition, while severe dysfunction is termed 'renal failure.' Renal stones may also occur through chronic dehydration.

Central nervous system

Seizures may occur secondary to electrolyte disturbances.

Psychological

Shame, guilt and disgust are common sequelae of vomiting and sufferers are often very secretive about this behaviour.

Medical and psychological consequences of binge eating

Weight gain and obesity

Binge eating even when associated with vomiting tends to lead to weight gain as most of the calories taken in are absorbed. In binge eating disorder where there are no compensatory mechanisms for weight gain, obesity may result.

Acute gastric dilatation/rupture/oesophageal rupture

This occurs more commonly in patients with bulimia nervosa but also occurs in patients with anorexia nervosa of the binge purge type and it may be rarely seen during refeeding. Gastric dilatation, if found to be chronic, may cause the stomach to lose contractibility, resulting in venous occlusion and possible gastric perforation (Figure 5.4). In the initial stages of treatment for this condition reversible changes may be possible, but as the disorder progresses irreversible damage to the gastric wall may occur. This is particularly so if large amounts are consumed after a long period of famine.

Psychological

Bingeing is commonly associated with marked emotional distress including feelings of guilt, shame, disgust and self-loathing.

Medical and psychological consequences of refeeding

Peripheral oedema

Peripheral oedema sometimes occurs in patients of low weight and is common during refeeding, especially in those who abuse laxatives.

Refeeding syndrome

Severe electrolyte and fluid shifts associated with metabolic abnormalities sometimes occur in malnourished patients undergoing refeeding, including abnormalities of fluid balance, glucose metabolism, hypophosphataemia, hypomagnesaemia, hypokalaemia and vitamin deficiency (Crook *et al.* 2001). The occurrence of hyophosphataemia may be reduced by commencing refeeding with a restricted (1500 Kcal daily) diet rich in phosphates (which are plentiful in dairy products).

Acute gastric dilatation/rupture

This may occur during refeeding but is rare. The occurrence may be minimized by commencing refeeding with a soft diet low in bulk.

Pancreatitis

This may occur with refeeding and raised amylase and abdominal pain may need to be distinguished from parotitis and refeeding pains (see above). Pancreatitis may also occur secondary to bingeing.

Psychological

Increased emotional distress and anxiety, especially around mealtimes is extremely common and this is sometimes managed with medication.

Conclusions

Patients with eating disorders require a thorough assessment of both medical and psychiatric risk with ongoing monitoring according to the clinical picture. Although the majority of the physical sequelae resolve with treatment of the eating disorder, some may require specific medical intervention. In these cases, it may be appropriate for general practitioners and psychiatrists managing patients with eating disorders to involve a physician with expertise in managing the physical consequences of eating disorders.

Further reading

Boyd C, Abraham S & Kellow K. Psychological features are important predictors of functional gastrointestinal disorders in patients with eating disorders. *Journal of Gastroenterology* 2005; **40**(8): 929–935.

Crook MA, Hally V & Panteli JV. The importance of refeeding syndrome. *Nutrition* 2001; **17**: 632–637.

Greenfeld D, Mickley D, Quinlan DM & Roloff P. Hypokalaemia in outpatients with eating disorders. *American Journal of Psychiatry* 1995; **152**(1): 60–63.

Herzog DB, Greenwood DN, Dorer DJ *et al.* Mortality in eating disorders: a descriptive study. *International Journal of Eating Disorders* 2000; **28**: 20–26.

Keilen M, Treasure T, Schmidt U & Treasure J. Quality of life measurements in eating disorders, angina and transplant candidates: are they comparable? *Journal of the Royal Society of Medicine* 1994; **87**: 441–444.

Keys A, Brozek J, Henschel A, Mickelson O & Taylor HL. *The Biology of Human Starvation.* University of Minnesota Press, Minneapolis, 1950.

Nielsen S, Møller-Madsen S, Isager T *et al.* Standardized mortality in eating disorders—a quantitative summary of previously published and new evidence. *Journal of Psychosomatic Research* 1998; **44**(3–4): 413–434.

Ogg EC, Millar HR, Pusztai EE & Thom AS. General practice consultation patterns preceding diagnosis of eating disorders. *International Journal of Eating Disorders* 1997; **22**(1): 89–93.

Rome ES & Ammerman S. Medical complications of eating disorders: an update. *Journal of Adolescent Mental Health* 2003; **33**: 418–426.

Sullivan PF. Mortality in anorexia nervosa. *American Journal of Psychiatry* 1995; **152**: 1073–1074.

Waldholtz BD & Andersen AE. Gastrointestinal symptoms in anorexia nervosa: a prospective study. *Gastroenterology* 1990; **98**: 1415–1419.

Wolfe BE, Metzger ED, Levine JM & Jimerson DC. Laboratory screening for electrolyte abnormalities and anaemia in bulimia nervosa: a controlled study. *International Journal of Eating Disorders* 2001; **30**: 288–291.

Zipfel S, Lowe B, Reas DL *et al.* Long-term prognosis in anorexia nervosa: lessons from a 21-year follow-up study. *The Lancet* 2000; **355**: 721–722.

CHAPTER 6

Comorbidity

Alex Yellowlees

OVERVIEW

- Comorbidity is important from both an academic and clinical perspective.
- Eating disorders have extensive psychiatric and physical comorbidity.
- It is vital to treat both psychiatric and physical comorbid conditions in their own right but also to be aware of the interactions.
- Physical and psychiatric comorbidity affect the response to treatment of the eating disorder.
- Depression, anxiety disorder, obsessive compulsive disorder, substance abuse and personality disorder are the most common psychiatric comorbid conditions.
- Significant family psychiatric comorbidity is also present in eating disorders.

What is comorbidity?

The concept of comorbidity is now well accepted in psychiatry and especially within the field of eating disorders. In this chapter it simply refers to the presence in patients of an eating disorder and one or more psychiatric or physical disorders occurring at the same time. The rate of psychiatric comorbidity in eating disorders is high and has been estimated to be between 70 and 90%. Affective disorders, anxiety disorders, obsessive compulsive disorder, substance abuse and personality disorders are the most commonly seen in clinical practice. It must be remembered that eating disorders can also occur in learning disability and psychosis where they may be easily overlooked.

Theoretically there is almost no medical condition which could not coexist with an eating disorder, and there are a few which must always be considered in the differential diagnosis—for instance thyroid conditions, wasting disorders and the side-effects of medications. However, one or two medical conditions in particular are notorious for their association with a poorer prognosis when comorbid with eating disorders. Diabetes mellitus is the most common of these, and cystic fibrosis, whilst less prevalent, is over-represented in eating disorders clinics.

ABC of Eating Disorders. Edited by J. Morris. © 2008 Blackwell Publishing, ISBN: 978-0-7279-1843-7.

How important is comorbidity?

Comorbidity in eating disorders is easily overlooked in clinical practice but is extremely important from a number of different perspectives. They include diagnosis, treatment, outcome, prognosis and research. The presence of a high degree of comorbidity may cause the actual validity of a diagnostic category itself to be questioned. It also raises important questions about the association between the conditions themselves and how they might influence each other. It can even yield vital information about the underlying causes and nature of eating disorders themselves.

In clinical terms, comorbidity is particularly relevant because it influences key areas of patient management, including:
- the course of the eating disorder;
- the treatments options to be considered;
- an individual's response to specific clinical interventions;
- the overall response to treatment;
- the prognosis.

What are the causes of comorbidity?

Chance is the simplest reason for the presence of comorbidity—common disorders simply co-occur more frequently. Another reason is sampling bias, which sometimes occurs in research studies in which greater levels of comorbidity are uncovered in patients selected from specialist eating disorder treatment units as compared to the general population.

Other possibilities include a high degree of sharing of risk factors and/or diagnostic criteria between a specific eating disorder and another psychiatric condition such as between that observed between obsessive compulsive disorder and anorexia nervosa, or bulimia nervosa and alcohol dependence for example. It has even been suggested that some eating disorders and comorbid psychiatric conditions could be different expressions of the same basic underlying physical and psychological pathology.

Psychiatric comorbidity

Family psychiatric comorbidity

High levels of psychiatric disorder are also found in the families of eating disorder sufferers, particularly in those with anorexia nervosa of the binge purge type and bulimia nervosa without a history

Table 6.1 Estimated lifetime prevalence rates for major depression as a comorbid condition in eating disorders.

Anorexia nervosa—restricting type	46–74%
Anorexia nervosa—binge/purge type	15–50%
Bulimia nervosa	50–60%
Binge eating disorder	46–58%

Table 6.2 Estimated lifetime prevalence rates for anxiety disorders as a comorbid condition in eating disorders.

Social phobias	20–59%
Specific phobias	15%
Panic disorder	11%
General anxiety disorder	10%

Table 6.3 Estimated prevalence rates for post-traumatic stress disorder as a comorbid condition in eating disorders.

Overall eating disorder population	13%
Bulimia nervosa	21%
Anorexia nervosa—restricting type	50%
Anorexia nervosa—binge/purge type	80%

Table 6.4 Estimated rates for childhood sexual abuse as a comorbid condition in eating disorders.

Anorexia nervosa	27%
Bulimia nervosa	51%
Binge eating disorder	30%

of previous anorexia. A positive family psychiatric history is often associated with more serious eating disorder symptoms and may carry a poorer prognosis for the patient.

Affective disorders

Mood disorder, particularly depression, is extremely common in individuals with eating disorders. Up to 75% of sufferers will experience a depressive illness over the course of their lifetime in contrast to only 10% a bipolar disorder (Table 6.1).

It is vital that the depression is identified and treated in its own right, using antidepressants and cognitive behavioural therapy (CBT).

Keep in mind too, that in anorexia nervosa the starvation state itself will negatively affect the response to medication and psychological therapy. Therefore the restoration of physical health to an adequate degree, including a healthier weight and high enough body mass index, is critical if the depressive condition itself is to improve.

Vomiting behaviour interferes with the absorption of antidepressant medication and it is imperative to direct patients to take their medication at a time of day when this negative effect will be minimized—usually as far removed as possible in time from the commencement of bingeing and vomiting, such as prior to sleep for example.

Anxiety disorders

Social withdrawal leading to reclusiveness and isolation commonly occurs as an eating disorder develops, particularly in anorexia nervosa. Patients may spend increasing amounts of time indoors, often in their bedroom, aside from when they may venture out in order to overexercise in a solitary way by walking or running.

The trademark phobic fears surrounding food and weight and the profound apprehension associated with eating along with others such as at family mealtimes or in restaurants with friends, are also commonplace.

However, in addition, specific anxiety disorders are frequently encountered in eating disorders. In anorexia and bulimia the lifetime prevalence for experiencing at least one anxiety disorder is about 70–80% and in binge eating disorder 9–46% (Table 6.2). These anxiety disorders should be managed with cognitive behavioural interventions along with standard pharmacological treatment.

Obsessional characteristics and obsessive compulsive disorder

Obsessive compulsive symptoms connected to food, exercise and weighing are frequently seen in eating disorder patients. But in addition a more distinct obsessive compulsive disorder (OCD) itself can often be detected. Obsessional personality characteristics in addition to OCD have been reported to occur in somewhere between 11–69% of women with anorexia nervosa and 3–43% of women with bulimia nervosa.

The actual lifetime prevalence of OCD has been estimated to be about 40% in eating disorder patients and is more commonly seen in anorexia nervosa compared to bulimia nervosa.

Patients should be treated with antidepressants, CBT and response prevention. Once again the response to treatment can be compromised by low weight and other comorbid conditions, and therefore improvement may take several years to occur in severe cases.

Post-traumatic stress disorder and childhood trauma

A history of childhood trauma is familiar among eating disorder sufferers, often as a result of physical or sexual abuse. Post-traumatic stress disorder (PTSD) can be a consequence. Estimated PTSD prevalence rates in eating disorder patients range from 13 to 80% (Table 6.3).

It has been suggested that childhood sexual abuse (CSA) is a non-specific risk factor for a range of psychiatric disorders, and elevated CSA rates are found in eating disorder patients (Table 6.4).

Substance abuse

Substance abuse in the form of alcohol or drug dependence is a problematic area of comorbidity, particularly in bulimia nervosa.

Table 6.5 Personality categories: estimated prevalence rates for personality clusters as a comorbid condition in eating disorders.

Personality clusters		AN (%)	BN (%)
A	Paranoid, schizoid and schizotypal	12	27
B	Narcissistic, borderline, antisocial and histrionic	15	44
C	Dependent, avoidant, obsessive-compulsive, passive aggressive	45	45
	Borderline alone	14	31

AN, anorexia nervosa; BN, bulimia nervosa.

Box 6.1 Vignette: Mandy

Mandy developed insulin-dependent diabetes at the 9 years of age and was encouraged by her middle-class parents to take pride in scrupulous injecting of insulin and 'perfectionistic' blood glucose control. By her teens she realised that she had gained weight as a result, and developed severe body image concern. Her sudden deterioration baffled her physicians but poor control was attributed to the onset of puberty and adolescent 'rebellion'. This was tolerated until alarming visual problems ensued and after some tearful interviews she was referred to the eating disorders clinic. Strangely, her chief motivation to change was distress about nocturia and recurrent thrush rather than concern about her eyesight.

Lifetime prevalence rates of substance use disorders have been reported to be 12–18% in anorexia nervosa and 30–70% in bulimia nervosa. These rates are very similar to the converse rates for eating disorders seen in alcohol dependence—anorexia nervosa 17%, bulimia nervosa 46%. In some cases it may be necessary to withdraw the patient from alcohol or drugs before attempting any significant eating disorder treatment; and referral to a specialist drug and alcohol service should be considered.

Personality disorder

A wide range of personality disorder types are well represented in bulimia nervosa but in anorexia nervosa dependant, avoidant, obsessive compulsive and passive aggressive types are the most commonly seen (Table 6.5). Borderline, narcissistic, histrionic and antisocial personality disorder categories are thought to be associated with poor treatment response and outcome.

Research has also identified three personality dimensional subtypes that intersect with eating disorder diagnoses:
- emotionally dysregulated and undercontrolled;
- high functioning and perfectionistic; and
- constricted and overcontrolled.

From a clinical perspective, personality disturbance influences the patient's presentation, capacity to engage in treatment, motivation, ability to sustain a therapeutic relationship, response to psychological intervention and likelihood of eventual recovery. It remains one of the most significant challenges in the management of eating disorder patients.

Physical comorbidity

Simulating conditions

A number of medical conditions can sometimes simulate eating disorders particularly if they produce unexplained weight loss or overeating.

Most commonly these are:
- malignancy;
- brain tumours;
- gastrointestinal disease; and
- acquired immunodeficiency syndrome (AIDS).

In general hospitals it is not uncommon to find eating disorders masquerading as other medical illnesses. Patients present with a wide range of signs and symptoms including unexplained weight loss, muscle weakness, abdominal pain, diarrhoea, constipation, amenorrhea, cardiac irregularities, anaemia, 'unstable' diabetes mellitus, epileptic seizures and even bone fractures due to osteoporosis.

Coexisting conditions

Eating disorders can be particularly difficult to manage when they co-occur with epilepsy, cystic fibrosis or diabetes mellitus. Patients taking anticonvulsant drugs may experience sedation and appetite changes leading to unwanted weight gain and body image distress. Attempts to minimize this using purging behaviours may result in electrolyte disturbances which exacerbate seizures and lead to the vicious circle of increased prescribing. In contrast, conditions such as cystic fibrosis and diabetes may themselves cause weight loss which, though pathological, is desirable to the patient, so that they are reluctant to adhere to prescribed diet and medication. It is always important to consider that patients with unstable or so called 'brittle' diabetes may be suffering from a coexisting but hidden eating disorder. In such situations it is well worth enquiring about the hallmark signs and symptoms of bingeing, fear of weight gain, preoccupation with shape and size, and body image distortion which can help to identify them and prompt consultation with liaison psychiatry or local eating disorder services. Symptoms such as vomiting, laxative abuse, calorie-counting and overexercise may be less prominent than in other eating disordered populations since under-use of insulin is a thoroughly effective weight-loss strategy on its own. It is also an extremely dangerous one and may lead to premature cardiovascular disease, neuropathies, end-stage kidney disease and blindness.

Body image concerns in the context of thyroid disorders may also lead patients to manipulate their medication, and those who are prescribed steroids may find themselves trapped in a vicious circle in which weight gain and 'moonface' cause embarrassment and distress whilst reducing the steroid dose leads to plummeting mood. These patients need sympathetic physicians to explicitly acknowledge their body image distress and discuss prescribing choices wherever possible.

Physical consequences

Physical comorbidity may reflect the extensive complications of weight loss and the serious consequences of bingeing and self-induced vomiting and laxative abuse. The metabolic, endocrine, dermatologic, gastrointestinal, cardiac, haematological, musculoskeletal and neurological systems are all involved. Along with suicide, such physical comorbidity makes a highly significant contribution to the very high mortality rate found in eating disorders. Chapter 5 provides more detail on the assessment and management of physical sequelae.

Further reading

Bellodi L, Cavallini MC, Bertelli S *et al*. Morbidity risk for obsessive-compulsive spectrum disorders in first-degree relatives of patients with eating disorders. *American Journal of Psychiatry* 2001; **158**(4): 563–569.

Bulik CM. Anxiety, depression and eating disorders. In: Fairburn CG & Brownell KD, eds. *Eating Disorders and Obesity*. Guilford Press, New York, 2002: 193–199.

Halmi KA, Eckert E, Marchi P *et al*. Comorbidity of psychiatric diagnosis in anorexia nervosa. *Archives of General Psychiatry* 1991; **48**: 712–718.

Milos GF. Axis I and II comorbidity and treatment experiences in eating disorder subjects. *Psychotherapy and Psychosomatics* 2003; **72**(5): 276–328.

Pearlstein T. Eating disorders and comorbidity. *Archives of Women's Mental Health* 2002; **4**: 67–78.

Rachelle L & Lilenfeld R. Psychiatric comorbidity associated with anorexia nervosa, bulimia nervosa, and binge eating disorder. In: Brewerton T, ed. *Clinical Handbook of Eating Disorders; an Integrated Approach*. Routledge, London, 2004: 183–184.

Woodside BD, Blake D & Staab R. Management of psychiatric comorbidity in anorexia nervosa and bulimia nervosa. *CNS Drugs* 2006; **20**(8): 655–663.

Zipfel S, Lowe B & Herzog W. Medical complications. In: Treasure J, Schimdt U & Furth E van, eds. *Handbook of Eating Disorders*, 2nd edn. John Wiley & Sons, Chichester, 2003: 169–190.

CHAPTER 7

What can a GP do? Management of Eating Disorders in Primary Care

Jane Morris and Nadine Harrison

OVERVIEW

- General practitioners (GPs) often struggle to find specialist care for eating disordered patients, or to persuade these patients to engage with such services.
- As the 'backstop' of care, GPs should avoid colluding with the anorexic drive to lose weight whilst providing unconditional physical monitoring, nurturing and risk assessment.
- The art of weighing a patient is delicate, fraught with deceptions and yet a valuable way both to monitor progress and understand distress.
- A dietician who is a specialist in eating disorders is a precious ally in the work with an anorexic patient. Anorexia usually 'runs rings round' dieticians who have no eating disorders experience.
- Patients with normal weight bulimia nervosa can be helped within primary care using high-dose selective serotonin reuptake inhibitors (SSRIs), advice on dietary behaviour and self-help materials.

This chapter and the next specifically focus on the role of the primary care team, and especially the GP. Physical and psychological management are separated only for convenience: integration of these aspects is essential.

A climate of sensitive and sensible awareness

At least 4% young women are affected by eating disorders, but even in areas where well-trained GPs have access to specialists, fewer than half are identified. Bulimia and binge eating disorder are roughly as common as (unipolar) depression. Low weight anorexia nervosa, though rarer, is as common in young women as psychotic illnesses.

In the early stages patients are protective of their eating disorder and avoid medical 'help'. People with anorexia fear weight gain. Overweight and even normal weight sufferers are handicapped by overwhelming body shame and the stigma attached to psychiatric diagnoses.

ABC of Eating Disorders. Edited by J. Morris. © 2008 Blackwell Publishing,
ISBN: 978-0-7279-1843-7.

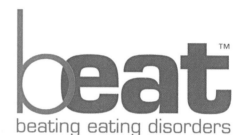

A UK wide charity providing information, help and support
for people affected by eating disorders including
anorexia and bulimia nervosa

beat Helpline 0845 634 1414
help@b-eat.co.uk
Open Monday to Friday 10:30am - 8:30pm
& Saturdays 1:00pm - 4:30pm

beat Youthline 0845 6347650
fyp@b-eat.co.uk
txt 07786 20 18 20
Open Monday to Friday 4:30pm - 8:30pm
& Saturdays 1:00pm- 4:30pm

www.b-eat.co.uk

beat is constantly developing its staff and as part of their training they may listen in to calls that are being taken by an experienced helpline worker
beat is a member of the Mental Health Helplines Partnership and abides by their guidelines

103 Prince of Wales Road, Norwich NR1 1DW
Admin T: 0870 770 3256 Media T: 0870 770 3221 F: 01603 664915
E: info@b-eat.co.uk

Figure 7.1 Beat poster for waiting room.

Compassionate awareness throughout the team must include receptionists and secretaries: it is also vital that any staff affected by eating disorders experience support and respect.

Posters and leaflets about eating disorders in the waiting room reassure patients that the practice does recognize their validity (Figure 7.1). The National Institute for Clinical Excellence (NICE) guidelines on eating disorders (NICE 2004) provide recommendations for professionals, and a clearly-written version for lay people. This should be made available to patients and their families at an early stage.

In most countries eating disorders are addressed by a patchwork of public, private and voluntary resources. There is often a struggle to find any resources at all. The Eating Disorders Association has a reliable directory of resources, and provides a lifeline (and phone line) for sufferers and carers.

The crucial therapeutic relationship

The GP is the ultimate backstop, the person to whom patients must be able to turn if therapy 'goes wrong'. Patients may not return unless the first disclosure of the eating disorder is met with kindness and commonsense. Beware, though, of 'walking on eggshells', failing to monitor weight or give robust advice for fear of 'scaring away' the patient.

Eating disorders may be conceptualized as a form of addiction. 'Motivational interviewing' encourages change (see Chapter 8). Motivation is not an all or nothing battle to be won before therapy can start, but an active strand throughout treatment. The guiding principle is to acknowledge and explore rather than fight the patient's ambivalence about recovery.

In even the best trials of eating disorders treatment, about 50% of patients fail to improve or drop out. These patients, for whom there is little evidence to guide management, remain the responsibility of general practice. Primary care staff need highly developed skills of acceptance, tolerance, resilient hope—and patient, persistent action.

What is helpful without becoming collusive?

The first priority is to distinguish a physically dangerous situation from one where there is time to negotiate. In a life-threatening emergency, hospitalization, however unpopular, is a sign of care and can ultimately enhance rather than jeopardize the therapeutic relationship. Doctors have legal and ethical responsibilities to prevent death or deterioration of health resulting from anorexia (see Chapter 11).

Outwith emergencies, wise doctors encourage patients to take as much responsibility for their own recovery as possible—'control' is a key component to such patients' sense of security. However, it is a doctor's duty both to provide all possible palliative and reparative care and to point out—without blaming or shaming—the associated damage. Eating disorders endanger patients and those around them. Doctors may need to offer unwelcome advice about refraining from sports and certain activities.

Binge-purging while driving is rarely disclosed unless you ask, and the risk of collapse also poses a greater hazard for drivers. Nursing shifts carry a risk of further disorder to body rhythms and lifting may precipitate stress fractures in an osteopenic spine. Emaciated children should not do physical education or use school as a pro-anorexic experience, but it is hard to remove a child's right to education unless parents and teachers understand the threat to health. Such issues can be compassionately rather than punitively acknowledged, and must be examined

rationally—discrimination against recovered sufferers is of course unwarranted and illegal.

When is it safe to keep care within the primary care team?

People who request specialist help for an eating disorder deserve the chance to use an evidence-based psychotherapy. Offer a 'stepped' approach (see Chapters 8 & 9) to those who are known to be of at least normal weight (body mass index [BMI] > 19 in adults). If the patient is reluctant, it is usually safe to refrain from specialist referral with a patient of normal weight. Medical emergencies are uncommon with bulimia or binge eating disorder, unless there are complications such as severe depression, self-harm or medical conditions such as diabetes, epilepsy or pregnancy.

At lower weight, refer unless weight is stable or rising, and take specialist advice about the urgency of the referral—clinics with long waiting lists prioritize emergencies, and may facilitate hospital admission. Weight instability, with frequent purging, compulsive exercise or comorbid substance abuse, is a stronger indicator for medical intervention than the actual BMI value.

Medical monitoring and attainment of a healthy stable weight

There are two contrasting approaches to anorexia:

1 For children and adolescents, where low weight threatens growth and development, refeeding comes first. Subsequent therapy helps patients tolerate and maintain normal weight. This approach is commonly used for adults too. Sadly, inpatient weight gain is rarely maintained without intensive outpatient follow-up.

2 A second approach temporarily accepts stable low weight while patients take responsibility for their own refeeding. Weight gain is slower, but more likely to be maintained, and with low iatrogenic risk.

Weighing without tears (Box 7.1)

Weight is of course the patient's own central concern. Calm, cheerful patients have often lost weight while an irritable or depressed mood may reflect the struggle to tolerate gain.

Doctors who do not weigh patients accurately, respectfully and cannily (as eating disorders dictate weight-distorting behaviours) are working in the dark and attract patients' secret scorn. Many patients 'falsify' weight with heavy objects, or 'water-loading' (a potential cause of pontine demyelination). It is helpful to acknowledge this, and make sure that weight loss is greeted with sympathy rather than disapproval.

Bullying patients onto the scales so that the doctor 'wins' and writes down a number in the records is likely to be counterproductive. Part of recovery is the ability to collaborate in accurate weekly weighing as our best—albeit still imperfect—monitor of changes in health and nutrition. Single weights tell us little. The construction and consideration of a weight graph is a therapeutic tool in itself (Figure 7.2). Weight gain is not synonymous with recovery,

Box 7.1 **How to weigh an outpatient with an eating disorder**

- Weighing is an intimate examination for someone with an eating disorder, and should be carried out respectfully, in privacy (**not** in a corridor or shared space) and using reliable, regularly calibrated scales.
- Aways try to weigh patients at the start of a session, not the end, as you may need time to digest the result together. There is rarely any point weighing more than once a week.
- It is usually acceptable to measure height—start with this, and in young patients repeat every 2 months.
- Ask if you may weigh the patient.
- If permission is declined, discuss as suggested in the text.
- If permission is given, agree to weigh the person on the same scales, in the same clothes and at the same time of day on each occasion. Suggest that the patient removes shoes, jackets and jumpers (this leaves 'light indoor clothes').
- Ask the patient to predict what the scales will say.
- Weigh the patient. **Do not comment on the result.**
- Record the result and plot this on a weight graph (or ask the patient to do this).
- Emphasize that a single point means very little—it takes three points on the graph to provide a meaningful trend. Ask the patient to comment on the slope of the graph.

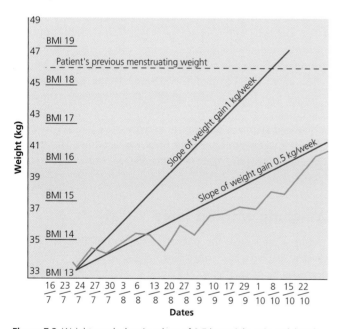

Figure 7.2 Weight graph showing slope of 0.5 kg weight gain and 'band' of normal weight range. BMI, body mass index.

but coming to terms with life without moving away from a healthy weight range is crucial.

Wise doctors discuss sleep, mood, concentration, libido, agitation, feeling the cold, interests and relationships—to demonstrate to the patient a broad concern for the quality of life rather than mirror their own pathological emphasis on weight. Patients belligerently confronted with medical investigations often resist change,

but encouragement in self-caring behaviour may gently steer them in the direction of recovery.

Essential physical care: responsible investigation without over investigation
(Figure 7.3 & Box 7.2)

Doctors who feel least confident in the management of eating disorders are most likely to search desperately for some 'medical' cause of weight loss. In children, neglect and abuse as well as medical syndromes should be considered, but the index of suspicion for anorexia nervosa as a cause of weight loss should be high in teenagers and young women. Making an early positive diagnosis of anorexia avoids long-winded searches for allergies, enzyme deficiencies or malignancies. Chapter 1 provides suggestions on responsible investigations (pp. 3 & 4).

Many abnormal results are expected in starvation—low white count should not trigger bone marrow biopsy, somewhat abnormal liver function tests (LFTs) are compatible with poor nutrition, low thyroid activity is actually cardioprotective at low weight. On the other hand, the fact that these result from starvation is no guarantee of safety—alcohol and paracetamol are even more toxic, low white count may still predispose to overwhelming infection, and low bone density to spinal collapse. Routine tests tell us little of intracellular changes—low serum potassium may reflect even lower intracellular levels of both potassium and magnesium, and the 'quick fix' of potassium supplements is largely cosmetic.

Referral to a dietician

Patients with normal weight bulimia nervosa are more likely to benefit from advice about structured eating *behaviour* than specifically nutritional advice. Patients can work through a list of principles of normal eating behaviour (Box 7.3).

Patients with anorexia benefit from *specialist* dietetic input. This needs to be in the context of family or therapeutic support, otherwise there is a tendency for the dietician to prescribe, while the patient simply fails to eat what is prescribed. Serfaty *et al.* (1999) were unable to compare cognitive behavioural therapy (CBT) with dietary advice in anorexia as all the dietary group dropped out of treatment!

An eating-disorders-trained dietician is the trusted expert who prescribes food scientifically, providing maximum nutritional value for calories, allowing health at the slimmest end of the normal weight range and demonstrating control of the weight graph. This allows carers to dismiss anorexic arguments about food, since the deal is that the dietician takes care of food prescribing.

Use of supplement drinks

Proprietary milkshake-type or fruit-juice-type boxed drinks cause controversy. Certainly they don't represent 'normal' social eating, but terrified ritualistic low-weight anorexic patients may be overwhelmed by the double task of taking in calories *and* adopting normal eating behaviours. Scientifically calculated food values are printed on each box so there is openness about what is prescribed

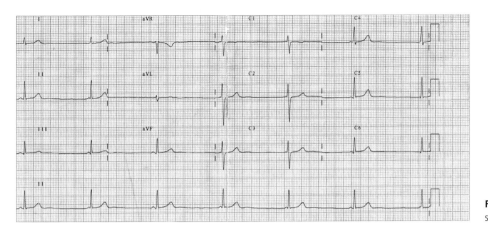

Figure 7.3 An electrocardiograph (ECG) showing bradycardia and hypokalaemia.

Box 7.2 **Recommended investigations (see also Chapter 1, p. 4)**

Bulimia nervosa
- Full physical examination is rarely needed, but blood tests may highlight low potassium, anaemia, and (in drinkers) abnormal liver function.

Anorexia nervosa
- The risk of overwhelming infection rises sharply when neutrophil count falls below 1×10/L. This is a useful rule of thumb, although there are probably other starvation-related factors contributing to susceptibility.

Box 7.3 **Principles of normal eating behaviour**

1 Aim for a balanced diet, including some of each main food group (protein, carbohydrate, fat) at every main meal.
2 Eat three meals and three snacks each day—evenly spaced eating prevents you from losing control through extreme starvation.
3 Aim to eat new and different foods. Make a list of your 'forbidden foods'—tick them off one by one as you manage them.
4 Chose normal food instead of 'low fat' or 'slimmer's' versions.
5 Write down what you eat in a diary.
6 Write in your diary the feelings or thoughts you experienced while you were eating or drinking, and afterwards, and any eating disordered behaviours you felt compelled to perform.
7 When possible, eat with other people rather than alone for a helpful perspective on normal eating, and a useful deterrent against binge/purging.
8 Explore ways to relax as much as possible before, during and after mealtimes—candles and nice tableware may help.
9 Plan your eating for at least the day ahead. Do not cram in too many activities during the day, but try not to have long periods of unstructured time either.
10 If you are in danger of binge/purging, plan what you will do at the end of each meal—leave the table or even the house.
11 Do not weigh yourself more than once a week—if possible let someone else, such as your doctor or therapist take over weighing.
12 When you find yourself 'feeling fat' make a note of the other difficulties in your life. Eating disorders make you feel anything painful in terms of feeling 'fat'.

---

and taken, and it may be healthier to use such drinks than eccentric unbalanced anorexic diets.

Further on in weight recovery, as metabolic rate shifts up a gear, it is hard to maintain a useful rate of weight gain without patients having to consume inconveniently large volumes of food. Here again, addition of a supplement drink is helpful and can later be discontinued to prevent undesirable overshoot beyond the intended weight.

Prescribing and the role of medication in eating disorders

For normal weight bulimia nervosa high dose antidepressants (e.g. fluoxetine 60 mg daily) offer proven but often short-lived antibulimic benefit (Walsh *et al.* 1991) even in the absence of overt depression, but benefits are inferior to the best psychological therapies (Agras *et al.* 1992).

Drug treatments are ineffective and potentially dangerous to starved patients (Kaye *et al.* 1991). There are a few exceptions: for prominent obsessive compulsive disorder symptoms high dose SSRIs may help even at low weight. Coexisting psychosis must of course be treated.

Contraceptive advice is essential for all sexually active patients regardless of weight. It is helpful when prescribing always to remember the high prevalence of undiagnosed bulimia. Patients who vomit need to know that the contraceptive pill takes up to an hour to be absorbed.

Further reading

NICE. *Eating Disorders: Core Interventions in the Treatment and Management of Anorexia Nervosa, Bulimia Nervosa and Related Eating Disorders.* NICE Clinical Guideline No 9. National Institute for Clinical Excellence, London, 2004: http://www.nice.org.uk

Strober M. Managing the chronic, treatment-resistant patient with anorexia nervosa. *International Journal of Eating Disorders* 2004; **36**(3): 245–255.

Walsh T, Hadigan C, Devlin M *et al.* Long-term outcome of antidepressant treatment for bulimia nervosa. *American Journal of Psychiatry* 1991; **148**: 1206–1212.

CHAPTER 8

Psychological Support within the General Practice

Jane Morris and Nadine Harrison

OVERVIEW

- Patients with eating disorders are ambivalent about recovery and may be enslaved by obsessive schedules and so benefit from extra tolerance within clinics and medical centres regarding such issues as lateness or non-attendances.

- Motivational enhancement interviewing techniques developed for use with substance misuse can also be useful in working with eating disorders.

- Parents and carers may be able to offer a helpful perspective which is not available from the patient. Living with someone with an eating disorder may be so painful that expression of emotion becomes destructive to all parties. Support for families may involve referral to self-help groups or outside support agencies to preserve boundaries.

- Common 'stuck points' can be anticipated and should be discussed within teams so that policies are evolved.

This chapter outlines the basics of a motivational approach, and considers further, more formal, 'psychological' interventions within primary care (Box 8.1). These will rarely fall to any but the most interested general practitioner (GP), although it will be the GP's role to assess whether patients can safely and usefully work with practice- or community-based counsellors and therapists, if available, or with relevant self-help materials, rather than referring to specialist facilities.

For the purposes of this chapter, the simple rule of thumb is that 'bulimia' refers to eating disordered patients of at least normal weight, while 'anorexia' refers to low weight patients. Most patients with normal or high weight bulimia or binge-eating disorders can be offered self-help or 'guided self-help' within primary care as a first intervention. Patients with stable anorexia nervosa may also accept low-key psychological support from primary care between episodes of more intensive treatment.

ABC of Eating Disorders. Edited by J. Morris. © 2008 Blackwell Publishing, ISBN: 978-0-7279-1843-7.

Box 8.1 **Case vignette: Jeannie**

Jeannie, a student teacher in her mid-20s, had disclosed details of her bulimia to her family general practitioner, Dr Brown, and was working through a self-help manual with the support and encouragement of the practice nurse. The receptionist asked Dr Brown if he would kindly 'pop through between patients' as Jeannie had become very distressed in the nurse's office.

Weekly weighing had revealed a 2 kg weight gain, after several weeks of weight stability and improvement in Jeannie's eating pattern. 'I knew this would happen if I gave up my diet, I can't trust the treatment if it is going to make me fat' she said, although by now she was no longer hysterical.

The nurse explained that Jeannie was at the stage of the treatment where she was managing not to make herself sick after binges. She was still unable to completely resist urges to binge although these were smaller than before. Both the nurse and the book Jeannie was following had explained at the start of therapy that people's weight usually increases a little at this stage but settles again by the end of treatment.

Dr Brown asked Jeannie to find the passage concerned with this in the self-help book and wondered whether she might consider alternatives to abandoning all her hard work at this stage. She agreed to tolerate the situation for 2 more weeks before returning to her previous weight control strategies. Happily, when she next returned her weight had fallen slightly and she reported that her period has started. She believed she had been 'water-retaining' as well as characteristically emotional the previous week.

Dr Brown suspected that the nurse had contrived his minimal intervention as a way to help the patient remain in the situation for long enough to let the anxiety diminish and to allow her to reflect on the best strategies rather than 'escape' into pathological behaviour without reflecting.

Awareness of motivational enhancement techniques

Patients do not eagerly seek relief from eating disorders in the same way as they might from physical disorders. Three important techniques help accommodate this ambivalence. The first is awareness of the cycles of readiness for change (Prochaska & Di Clemente) (Figure 8.1).

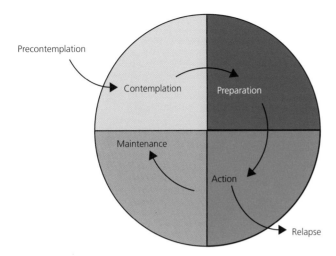

Figure 8.1 Transtheoretical model—stages of change. Motivation for change is considered to fall within one of the illustrated stages of readiness for change. *Precontemplation* the person sees no benefit in change—s/he does not regard the issue as a problem to be solved. The stage of *Contemplation* is one of ambivalence, and the individual is aware of the possibility and even desirability of change, but is also aware of the difficulties, disadvantages and dangers of attempting change. *Preparation*—the patient often needs to do a great deal of thinking and planning before there can be any *Action*. *Maintenance* is crucial—most change requires hard work to be maintained to deal with lapses, before they become full-blown *Relapses*. Lasting recovery normally includes the experience of surviving several relapses.

People may move between different stages in the course of a day (or an hour), and be in different stages for different behaviours—a patient may wish to change their bingeing, vomiting and laxative abuse, but be ambivalent about exercise addiction, and be in a precontemplative stage with regard to remaining as thin as possible. Families and carers are often in the *Action* or even *Maintenance* stage while patients remain in precontemplation or at best contemplative stage, so that once the patient leaves her family's care, she loses weight again.

Adult patients with bulimia nervosa rarely consult a doctor before they have mustered considerable motivation for change—although the change they seek is sometimes for more effective weight-loss techniques rather than psychological and physical help. They are usually in the 'contemplation' or 'preparation' stages of readiness for change (see Figure 8.1). Once embarked on treatment, success often breeds further success, especially when using cognitive behavioural therapy (CBT).

It is harder to engage those with anorexia. Early in the disorder symptoms feel more like solutions than problems; later on anorexia becomes the patient's whole identity—the prospect of relinquishing it is terrifying. They remain in the 'precontemplation' (see Figure 8.1) stage of readiness for change. The technique of 'separating the person from the disorder' may seem merely a politically correct way of speaking, but in fact it does help the doctor to sympathize with patients without colluding with the disorder that preys on their health. It is more acceptable to say, 'Mary I see that anorexia is forcing you to run to school when we agreed you'd use the bus.' than to accuse her of flouting your advice.

The third technique of the trio is the art of 'motivational interviewing'—incorporating a battery of listening and questioning

---

Box 8.2 **Principles of motivational interviewing**

Anticipate ambivalence

You cannot expect patients to 'really want to change'. Encourage patients to gather information from reputable books, leaflets, the internet, and from their physical investigation results and reported symptoms, so that they can identify both the disadvantages of eating disordered behaviour and perceived advantages. They will struggle to give up the advantages unless other ways can be found to supply these.

Express empathy

An eating disorder is a misfortune not a crime! Use open-ended questions and reflective listening skills; do not constantly 'steamroll' what is said with your own 'buts'. Most doctors talk more than they listen. People are more likely to believe and act upon ideas that come out of their own mouths!

Roll with resistance

If you notice you have got into a fight so that you feel you are attacking the eating disorder and they are defending it, STOP! Acknowledge this and make up. Agree to both be on the side of the patient's greatest good; even if at present you make different assumptions about what this involves.

Support self-efficacy

Maintain hope, and show that you believe recovery *is* possible. Endorse and encourage the patient's intentions and efforts in the direction of recovery. Point out other areas of life in which the patient has been successful. Help the patient draw up their own realistic programme for change, identifying tailor-made goals and possible techniques. Personal control is particularly important to someone with an eating disorder.

Caution: In practice none of us has the choice not to eat, and life-threateningly ill patients need you to take away control and make choices for them—it is crucial to recognize such situations and be clear about your medical duty. Handing back control gradually is then an essential part of therapy. It is often helpful to ask patients, 'Who is making this choice—you or anorexia'?

---

skills to develop and enhance the patient's readiness to fight the anorexia (Box 8.2). The constant rebuilding of motivation feels like painting the Forth Bridge. It is essential to remember that recovery usually takes 3–6 years, and may even occur after more than two decades of apparently 'chronic' anorexia.

Keeping patients engaged in treatment (Box 8.3)

Anorexia causes people to be unduly concerned with appearances (Figure 8.2), so these patients find it extraordinarily painful not to 'look good.' They want professionals to be pleased with them but desperately succumb to 'anorexic rules' too. Weight loss risks the doctor's disapproval while weight gain disobeys the anorexia and provokes guilt, fear and fury. One option is to 'fake' weight gain, another is to fail to turn up.

Box 8.3 **Outline of basic psychological management**

- Before attempting any change, both parties discuss their concept of the eating disorder and draw up collaborative goals of treatment. Baselines are recorded—questionnaires, height and weight, perhaps a week's food diary.
- A contract is drawn up with practical arrangements for the course of treatment.
- Psycho-education is a motivational preparation—the patient uses books, leaflets, the internet, discussion and other means to explore what is known about the eating disorder—causes, consequences and treatments.
- Change starts with straightforward behavioural work—patients try to act on as many as possible of the 'principles of normal eating behaviour'. At this stage there is no expectation to address binge-purge behaviours.
- Once the basic healthy eating pattern is in place, patients gradually dispense with pathological behaviours—binge-purging, obsessive weighing or body-checking, compulsive exercise. At this stage cognitive techniques are introduced—identifying and challenging disordered assumptions. This can be done by questioning the truth of them theoretically and by 'behavioural experiments' designed to test them out in reality.
- Residual emotional issues are considered—assertiveness, interpersonal issues, depression, anxiety, trauma and abuse. These may require further referral. Healthy eating makes the brain better able to use psychotherapy, and success in overcoming the eating disorder encourages the patient in further work.

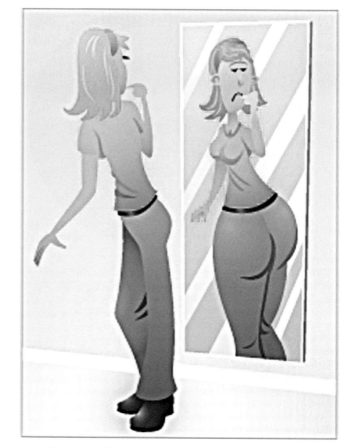

Figure 8.2 Repeated critical scrutiny of one's reflection leads to perceptual distortion and to the vicious circle of further search for reassurance that the body is not fat or misshapen.

Patients with normal weight bulimia often miss appointments out of embarrassment (Figure 8.3). If they show a food diary detailing disgusting binge–purge episodes, they will feel mortified. If they withhold the evidence they have failed to do their 'homework', so it is simpler to break the appointment.

No-shows are met with understandable disapproval in busy practices. Patients may drop out altogether rather than face an angry receptionist. Expectations of motivation and appointment-keeping which are appropriate to patients with medical and surgical needs are unrealistic for those with psychological disorders and particularly eating disorders.

Attendance difficulties should be explicitly anticipated. A course of appointments can be set up in advance with the agreement that one missed meeting does not constitute dropout. Regular attendance for monitoring and discussion can be spelled out as an important goal of treatment rather than a presumption.

Regular assertive follow up for chronically anorexic patients need not amount to regular therapy. Left alone, under half of them remain in touch with services, but centres offering low-key monitoring with occasional brief crisis interventions report half the mortality and increased eventual recovery rates.

The role of guided self-help, supported by practice staff

Chapter 9 describes self-help in more detail. This chapter examines the role of primary care staff in prescribing and supporting the use of available materials.

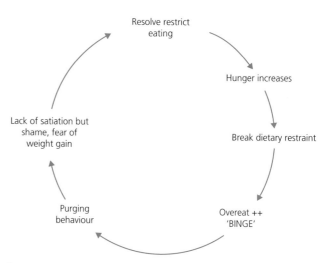

Figure 8.3 The vicious circle of bulimia nervosa. The more extreme the restraint and purging, the more urgent and enormous the overeating episodes, which in turn drive more frantic weight-control attempts.

Some familiarity with the rationale for and outline of the main evidence-based approaches allows better integration of the materials into the patient's care. For patients, an interested professional to monitor progress reinforces motivation—rather like adding the benefits of an occasional driving lesson to the New Year resolution to learn to drive, even if an intensive course is not available.

Manuals can be administered by minimally trained professionals or offered in workbook form as 'self-help'. It is less stigmatizing for patients to attend their local medical practice, and many areas have minimal specialist facilities for any but the most severely affected patients. Guided self-help can also be educational for the professional involved. Working alongside a bulimic patient, guided by a clearly written self-help book teaches the knowledge base in the field of eating disorders; provides an overview of the guiding principles of CBT; and offers the live experience of therapy in action. Patients can benefit from meeting a therapist as infrequently as every 4 or 6 weeks, either individually or in group format.

Benefit from self-help is strongly correlated with outcome in formal CBT. Both approaches rely heavily on patients' capacity for self-monitoring—the mainstay of CBT for bulimia nervosa (CBT-BN) is the 'food diary', listing food intake, binge-purge episodes and associated feelings and thoughts (Figure 8.4). Some patients will make considerable progress with self-help materials but still benefit from referral for formal CBT to achieve fuller recovery. Those who experience only failure with CBT-based models may prefer specific referral for interpersonal psychotherapy (IPT) where this is available.

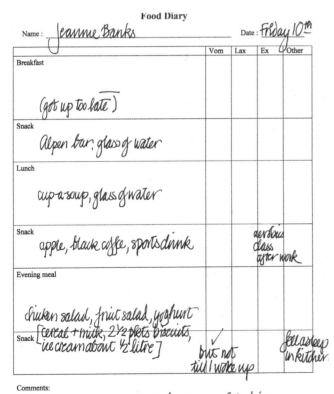

Figure 8.4 Food diary with thoughts and comments.

Support for families and carers

Younger patients and those with low weight anorexia of whatever age are likely to be brought to treatment by their families. Positive family involvement is a powerful resource, but the stresses of living with someone with anorexia make some relatives behave in unhelpful ways. The ideal attitude for all carers, whether family or professional, is firm and non-collusive, but very calm. Support networks, including support groups and help-lines can keep carers' own emotional health and morale up to the marathon task of facilitating recovery.

Professionals who hear only the patient's side of the story may offer insufficient help or credence to the family, and be insufficiently firm with the patient themselves. This is a common form of unrecognized collusion. Conversely, failure to understand the imperatives of an eating disorder can result in the view that patients are merely naughty or selfish and undeserving of treatment. The role of the family is considered further in Chapter 13.

Common stuck points and how to tackle them

Refusal to accept diagnosis

Diagnosis validates the right to effective treatment and provides colleagues with important information. You may, though, agree with the patient to make use of less offending terms such as 'your eating' or 'your weight concern' in conversations. Ask why the patient dislikes the diagnostic label—some are afraid it compels them to have treatment, some protect their eating disorder from change by conceptualizing it as something else (allergy, Candida, bowel disease), some fear the stigma of a psychiatric disorder.

Refusal to be weighed

Do not give up on the effort to monitor weight any more than you would give up on the effort to monitor blood sugar in a diabetic patient.

If an emaciated patient refuses to be weighed, point out that in the absence of a reliable weight graph, decisions about hospitalization and management must be based on a pessimistic estimate of weight trends.

Complaints about quality of food

Food is medicine for eating disorders. It does not have to taste wonderful. No-one was ever 'tempted better' by gourmet food!

Vegetarianism, veganism and religious food restriction

Refeeding diets can accommodate vegetarian guidelines, but cannot usually safely exclude all animal products. Most refeeding programmes ask patients to relax veganism to vegetarianism until a healthy weight is achieved. It may emerge that the dietary restriction originated in anorexia rather than in moral or religious belief—the patient can take back moral responsibility for the choice when health is restored. Religious advisors are usually glad to provide official dispensation from fasting or extreme dietary practices if these affect the believer's health.

Patient refuses permission to talk to family

Eating disorders, like any form of self-harm, may threaten life and health. When the danger is acute, carers (lay or professional) need to know enough to keep the patient safe. You should not disclose any information beyond this minimum until the patient feels enough trust and desire to enlist the further support of the family—this is to be welcomed, not imposed. Patients who refuse permission to disclose their weight may allow the shape of the weight graph to be shared, but with the numbers covered.

Exercise dependence

Patients rarely complain of their exercise dependence, but GPs do well to ask about it. Insist that fragile low-weight patients stay warm and avoid bone stress (no skiing!). Encourage yoga and tai chi to replace high-impact exercise. Professionals should not make the mistake of condoning compulsive activity that does not result in weight loss—it can be a severe problem in itself. Patients need to learn that rest and relaxation are positive reparative skills, not 'laziness'.

'Multi-impulsive' eating disorders with self-harm and substance misuse

Chaotic bulimia may be just one of a range of self-harming behaviours in sufferers who also meet criteria for borderline disorder. They may benefit from dialectical behavioural therapy (DBT) or dynamic psychotherapy—straightforward CBT-BN is less likely to be effective. At low weight, substance misuse, purging and other forms of self-harm are all far more lethal and there should be a much lower than normal threshold for referring the patient for emergency medical attention. General practitioners do their best to monitor physical safety, but therapy is beyond the scope of primary care.

Further reading

Cooper PJ. *Bulimia Nervosa and Binge-eating: A Self-help Guide.* Robinson, London, 1993.

Fairburn CG. *Overcoming Binge Eating.* Guilford Press, New York, 1995. *(**This self-help manual is very similar to Cooper's (above) and addresses bulimia nervosa as well as non-purging binge disorders. It includes an excellent summary of theory and research in straightforward language—highly recommended for professionals as well as more sophisticated patients.**)*

Strober M. Managing the chronic, treatment-resistant patient with anorexia nervosa. *International Journal of Eating Disorders* 2004; **36**(3): 245–255.

Treasure J & Schmidt U. *Clinician's Guide to Getting Better Bit(e) by Bit(e): A Survival Kit for Sufferers of Bulimia Nervosa and Binge Eating Disorders.* Psychology Press, Sussex, 1997.

Treasure J & Ward A. A practical guide to the use of motivational interviewing in anorexia nervosa. *European Eating Disorders Review* 1997; **5**: 102–114.

CHAPTER 9

Advice, Education and Self-help

Chris Williams and Ulrike Schmidt

OVERVIEW

- Self-help gives the person control over how and when they work, and is also especially helpful where shame, anxiety, low confidence or guilt would otherwise prevent the person engaging.

- Of the evidence-based treatments for eating disorders, cognitive behavioural therapy (CBT) stands out as the therapy that can most easily be delivered as self-help, and is also the best-evidenced treatment for bulimia nervosa.

- Interventions can be offered using a variety of media—CBT self-help books, websites, CD-ROMs and possibly other self-help formats such as DVDs.

- Self-help for eating disorders should not overlook the fact that medical risk issues may need to be addressed.

- Unfortunately websites vary from being helpful, accurate sources of reputable information, through to those that are poorer or misleading in content, to the potentially harmful 'pro-ana' sites.

- Informational and self-help approaches are not 'magic' answers but offer a sensible way for services to increase their capacity to offer treatment.

Introduction

Eating disorders are common disorders, affecting mainly adolescents and young adults. On reviewing the effective treatments for eating disorders (NICE 2004), two forms of therapy stand out:

- cognitive behavioural therapy (CBT) for bulimia nervosa and binge-eating disorders;
- family-based/systemic approaches for adolescents with anorexia nervosa.

Unfortunately, the number of trained and accredited practitioners available who are expert in either therapeutic model is limited. For example, it is clearly not possible to offer 12–20 one-to-one hour-long sessions of specialist CBT to every patient. Given the increasing need for treatment, a major challenge is therefore to adapt CBT to make it more widely available.

ABC of Eating Disorders. Edited by J. Morris. © 2008 Blackwell Publishing, ISBN: 978-0-7279-1843-7.

A second challenge is the reluctance of people with eating disorders to seek professional help. This is partly an age-related phenomenon, as adolescents and young adults are generally reluctant to seek help from professional sources (Oliver *et al.* 2005) and prefer self-help approaches over and above therapist-led interventions (Jorm *et al.* 2004). Moreover, disorder-specific factors may make engagement with health services difficult for a proportion of people with eating disorders. Thus in anorexia nervosa sufferers themselves value their disorder and underestimate or down-play the risks, whereas their parents and other carers are usually desperate for information and practical advice about how to help their child. People with bulimia nervosa or binge eating disorder are often ashamed about their bingeing and weight control practices, and may therefore avoid seeking help, resulting in high levels of hidden morbidity. Having up-to-date, relevant information that facilitates viewing one's problems in a new and different light may help improve motivation to change for those who are reluctant to, especially if such information is easily accessible and presented in a user-friendly format.

Self-help approaches

One solution to the challenge presented by limited therapeutic resources is to offer access to expert psychological therapy delivered in ways other than having to see a practitioner for one-to-one work, e.g. through translating a programme of therapy into a self-help format. The term self-help is used to describe, 'The delivery of materials that employ a media based format to treatment such as book, computer or video tape. However delivered, self-help materials aim to increase the user's knowledge about a particular problem, and also to equip them with skills to better self-manage their difficulties' (Williams 2003). Self-help treatments may be provided independently from (unsupported self-help) or in addition to (supported or guided self-help) sessions with a health care practitioner.

Of the evidence-based treatments for eating disorders, CBT stands out as the therapy which can most easily be delivered as self-help. This is because:

- It has a structure and psycho-educational focus that translates well into books or computer programs.
- Much of the efficacy of CBT is the step by step approach it utilizes to help people understand why they feel as they do, and then learn

new life skills they can use in their own lives. The idea of CBT being a self-help form of therapy is central to this approach.

- Many CBT practitioners utilize CBT self-help materials to supplement therapy sessions. Here, the materials help take forward the therapy between face-to-face sessions, as well as providing a permanent reminder of what has been learned to date.
- It is flexible—it allows the person to work on their problems at a pace, time and place they wish.
- CBT self-help is particularly suited to eating disorders because it gives the person control over how and when they work. It is also especially helpful where shame, anxiety, low confidence or guilt (Burney & Irwin 2000) would otherwise prevent the person engaging.

There is now a growing evidence base that CBT interventions can be offered in different ways such as using CBT self-help books, websites, CD-ROMs and possibly other self-help formats such as DVDs (e.g. http://www.livinglifetothefull.com). Such developments have been slower to be developed in eating disorders than in some other disorders such as anxiety and depression, most likely because of the medical risk issues involved.

Evidence base for self-help in eating disorders

Over recent years, a string of recommendations have been made for CBT self-help to be introduced into clinical services as part of so-called *stepped care approaches*. This suggests that simpler, accessible treatments are offered first. The National Institute for Clinical Excellence (NICE) guidelines for eating disorders (NICE 2004) suggested that structured self-help approaches based on CBT models can be a useful first step for the treatment. A recent Cochrane review has confirmed that CBT self-help is a good first step to therapy for bulimia nervosa—but that the evidence base for self-help is currently lacking for anorexia nervosa (Perkins *et al.* 2006).

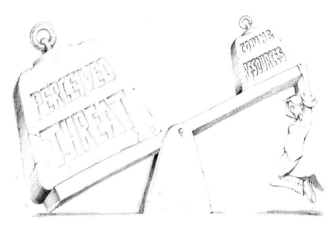

Figure 9.1 Cognitive behavioural therapy (CBT) interventions try to teach new coping resources and help get problems in perspective. (Figure drawn by Keith Chan; reproduced with permission.)

Books/bibliotherapy

Bibliotherapy refers to the use of written self-help materials. Almost all studies to date have utilized CBT. Several written manuals have been shown to be effective in the treatment of bulimia nervosa and binge eating disorder. For example:

- *Getting Better Bite by Bite* (Schmidt & Treasure 1993; example research paper: Treasure *et al.* 1996).
- *Overcoming Binge Eating* (Fairburn 1995; example research paper: Palmer *et al.* 2002).

The approach offers the prospect of significant savings in clinical support, thereby increasing the capacity of services to help. For example, Thiels *et al.* (1998) using *Getting Better Bite by Bite* (translated into German) found that there was no significant difference in outcome between eight fortnightly sessions plus the book compared to 16 weekly individual sessions of CBT. Here, dropout, rate, general satisfaction with treatment and views regarding the usefulness of the therapies were identical in the two treatment groups (but interestingly not by some other local practitioners—see later).

Computerized cognitive behavioural therapy (CCBT)

If books can be helpful, can similar information be delivered in other ways? For example in depression a recent major review of the field has confirmed that materials in book form are no more or less effective than those delivered by computer (e.g. CD-ROMs or online programs—Gellatly *et al.* 2007). Therefore, it is likely that self-help treatments can be offered via the computer. In fact there may be several advantages to this. For example, multimedia approaches may make things seem more personal (e.g. seeing a video of someone) and immediate. There is also the possibility of making the program interactive—asking questions and providing specific responses based on the answers given.

In other settings such as anxiety and depression, CCBT is now recommended by NICE (e.g. NICE 2006). A number of new computer-based packages have been developed to address eating disorders including the Salut Guide (http://www.salut-ed.org/) and Overcoming Bulmina Online (http://www.overcomingbulimiaonline.com) for people with bulimia and eating disorders not otherwise specified, and Overcoming Anorexia Online (http://www.overcominganorexiaonline.com) aimed at carers of those with anorexia.

Several free websites make available interventions for low mood, prevention of depression and free life skills training—all with a CBT focus. These might well also be of help for people with eating disorders to address general problems such as anxiety, and how to tackle negative thinking, problem solving, avoidance and depression. Two sites that are widely used are:

- Mood Gym (http://moodgym.anu.edu.au/). This aims to help prevent depression, and provides a detailed cognitive behaviour therapy treatment package.
- Living Life to the Full (http://www.livinglifetothefull.com). This site run by the author (Chris Williams) provides information, teaching resources, mood rating, a self-help forum and free life skills packages and receives over a million 'hits' a month.

Online computerized resources for eating disorders

Online resources include blogs, wikis, support forums, information sources, special interest pages run by individuals (e.g. who have experienced eating problems) as well as popular voluntary sector sites. Two well-known and widely recommended sites are:

- Institute of Psychiatry (http://www.iop.kcl.ac.uk/iop/Departments/PsychMed/EDU/index.shtml);
- Beat (formally the Eating Disorders Association) (http://www.b-eat.co.uk/Home), which receives over 3 million 'hits' a month.

Unfortunately websites vary from being helpful, accurate sources of reputable information, such as those above, through to those that are poorer or misleading in content. Some sites to be especially aware of that could potentially be harmful to patients are so-called 'pro-ana' sites. These encourage users to lose weight and provide reinforcement to do so. This is a concern in view of the significant growth of available sites addressing eating disorders online and the potential power of others reinforcing unhelpful beliefs and behaviours and urging ever further weight loss.

Support and self-help

In depression there has been a clear finding that adding in support from a practitioner or other worker (not necessarily qualified) significantly improves the outcome of the patient/client (Gellatly *et al.* 2007). It would be expected that this would be also the case in bulimia—yet one published paper has suggested no benefits of adding support (Murray *et al.* 2007). However, the sample was small and the result could reflect a study that was simply underpowered. For the time being it therefore seems sensible to provide support. It appears that telephone support is as effective as face-to-face support (e.g. Palmer *et al.* 2002; Gellatly *et al.* 2007). Other support types that may be effective but have not been investigated sufficiently are email, live chat, videoconferencing and using moderated forum support.

Problems when it comes to introducing self-help into services

A major issue here is that it takes:

(a) time to make changes in service design; and
(b) enthusiasm for such change.

Many practitioners have doubts that self-help approaches can be useful. They may be happy to agree that providing information is useful; however, they may have concerns that using CBT self-help to provide some of the therapy (or even as an alternative to therapy) will result is something '*second-best*' being offered. Some practitioners who have introduced self-help have encountered scepticism amongst some colleagues (e.g. Thiels 2005; Hitchcock, unpublished MSc thesis).

Perhaps here the questions being asked are the wrong ones. Instead of assuming we 'know' a particular therapy is best, we should instead be asking, 'What do people need—including those I am not seeing because our service is not addressing their needs'? Overall guided CBT self-help is about as effective as seeing a therapist. This is true of books (e.g. Bailer *et al.* 2005; Schmidt *et al.* 2007) and computerized delivery (e.g. Bara-Carril *et al.* 2004).

We also know that in depression the provision of information alone is simply not as effective as CBT self-help (Gellatly *et al.* 2007), yet it appears that it is the latter (effective) treatment that causes practitioners the most concern. It is also known that attitudes towards the use of CBT self-help change for the positive when practitioners have training in using the approach (Whitfield & Williams 2004).

Such change is important because services—and a lack of services—are currently failing people. We know that there is a significant *treatment gap* between the proportion of people with eating disorders and the number of people receiving treatments in services (e.g. Treasure *et al.* 2005). This gap is the result of various factors including stigma, fear, lack of confidence, lack of knowledge, poor communication and links between compartmentalized services, as well as a crucial lack of provision of services in ways that people can access them.

Perhaps this therefore is the challenge of stepped care models. It is not an issue of information *or* self-help *or* one-to-one treatments. All are needed in services. Instead matched assessment based on patient need and preference is required to provide services acceptable and local to the patient. Services should be designed with the person in mind. This includes outreach work to places where people with eating disorders are (such as schools, dentists, youth clubs), including a range of ways of accessing help (not just one to one—which may scare off some people from seeking help). This could include providing options such as working through written CBT self-help books, or using computerized and quality online resources to begin work. Support might be offered by National Health Service workers or others such as voluntary sector workers to broaden inclusion. Provision of links to quality support sites such as the Beat website should be encouraged.

Summary and conclusions

Someone once said 'information is power'. Informational and self-help approaches are important and hold much promise. They are not however 'magic' answers. They should be neither rejected out of hand, nor made too important in services. Instead they offer a sensible way for services to increase their capacity to offer treatment. They are useful additions to resources, and crucially can offer a useful first step to treatment that draws people towards accepting effective help that so many currently fail to receive.

Further reading

Bailer U, de Zwaan M, Leisch F *et al.* Guided self-help versus cognitive-behavioral group therapy in the treatment of bulimia nervosa. *International Journal of Eating Disorders* 2004; **35**: 522–537.

Bara-Carril N, Williams CJ, Pombo-Carril MG *et al.* A preliminary investigation into the feasibility and efficacy of a CD-ROM based cognitive-behavioural self-help intervention for bulimia nervosa. *International Journal of Eating Disorders* 2004; **35**: 538–548: http://www3.interscience.wiley.com/cgi-bin/fulltext/108068602/PDFSTART

Bower P & Gilbody S. Stepped care in psychological therapies: access, effectiveness and efficiency. Narrative literature review. *British Journal of Psychiatry* 2005; **186**: 11–17.

Burney J & Irwin HJ. Shame and guilt in women with eating-disorder symptomatology. *Journal of Clinical Psychology* 2000; **56**: 51–61.

Fairburn CG. *Overcoming Binge Eating*. Guilford Press, New York, 1995.

Gellatly J, Bower P, Hennessy S *et al*. What makes self-help interventions effective in the management of depressive symptoms? Meta-analysis and meta-regression. *Psychological Medicine* 2007; **37**: 1217–1228.

Jorm AG, Griffiths KM, Christensen H *et al*. Actions taken to cope with depression at different levels of severity: a community survey. *Psychological Medicine* 2004; **34**: 293–299.

Murray K, Schmidt U, Pombo-Carril M-G *et al*. Does therapist guidance improve uptake, adherence and outcome from a CD-ROM based cognitive-behavioral intervention for the treatment of bulimia nervosa? *Computers in Human Behavior* 2007; **23**(1): 850–859: http://dx.doi.org/10.1016/j.chb.2004.11.014

NICE. Computerised cognitive behaviour therapy for depression and anxiety. *Review of Technology Appraisal* 2006; **51**: http://www.nice.org.uk

NICE. *Eating Disorders: Core Interventions in the Treatment and Management of Anorexia Nervosa, Bulimia Nervosa and Related Eating Disorders*. NICE Clinical Guideline No 9. National Institute for Clinical Excellence, London, 2004: http://www.nice.org.uk

Oliver MI, Pearson N, Coe N & Gunnell D. Help-seeking behaviour in men and women with common mental health problems: cross-sectional study. *British Journal of Psychiatry* 2005; **186**: 297–301.

Palmer RL, Birchall H, McGrain L *et al*. Self-help for bulimic disorders: a randomised controlled trial comparing minimal guidance with face-to-face or telephone guidance. *British Journal of Psychiatry* 2002; **181**: 230–235.

Perkins SJ, Murphy R, Schmidt U & Williams C. Self-help and guided self-help for eating disorders. *Cochrane Database of Systematic Reviews* 2006; **3**: CD004191. DOI: 10.1002/14651858.CD004191.pub2.

Schmidt U & Treasure J. *Getting Better Bite by Bite*. Lawrence Erlbaum Associates, East Sussex, Hove, 1993.

Schmidt U, Lee S, Beecham J *et al*. A randomized controlled trial of family therapy and cognitive behavior therapy guided self-care for adolescents with bulimia nervosa and related disorders. *American Journal of Psychiatry* 2007; **164**: 591–598.

Thiels C, Schmidt U, Treasure J *et al*. Guided self-change for bulimia nervosa incorporating use of a self-care manual. *American Journal of Psychiatry* 1998; **155**: 947–953.

Treasure J, Schmidt U & Hugo P. Mind the gap: service transition and interface problems for patients with eating disorders. (Editorial) *British Journal of Psychiatry* 2005; **18**(7): 398–400.

Treasure J, Schmidt U, Troop N *et al*. Sequential treatment for bulimia nervosa incorporating a self care manual. *British Journal of Psychiatry* 1996; **168**: 94–98.

Whitfield G & Williams CJ. If the evidence is so good why doesn't anyone use them? Current uses of computer-based self-help packages. *Behavioural and Cognitive Psychotherapy* 2004; **32**(1): 57–65.

Williams C. New technologies in self-help: another effective way to get better? (Editorial) *European Eating Disorders Review* 2003; **11**: 170–182: http://www3.interscience.wiley.com/cgi-bin/fulltext/104528308/PDFSTART

Acknowledgements

Conflict of interest statement: Dr Chris Williams is author of the websites Living Life to the Full (http://www.livinglifetothefull.com) and Overcoming Bulimia Online (http://www.overcomingbulimia-online.com), and Professor Ulrike Schmidt and Dr Chris Williams are amongst the authors of the website Overcoming Anorexia Online (http://www.overcominganorexiaonline.com).

CHAPTER 10

Specialist Referral

Jon Arcelus and Bob Palmer

OVERVIEW

- Most established eating disorders warrant referral to secondary or tertiary care services.
- The National Institute for Clinical Excellence (NICE) guideline sets out what should usually be offered to people with eating disorders.
- Specialist eating disorder services for adults are growing in numbers but are still patchy and some services are limited in what they can provide.
- Most child and adolescent mental health services (CAMHS) treat eating disorders as part of their core remit.
- The transition from CAMHS to adult services can be problematic.

Some general practitioners (GPs) and other primary care workers have sufficient experience and expertise to manage with confidence many of their eating disordered patients solely in primary care. Most do not. For the majority of cases of established eating disorder (ED) it is sensible to involve clinicians who do have such expertise. This means making a referral to some sort of 'specialist' in secondary or tertiary services (Box 10.1). However, after referral the primary care team may still play key roles in complex care plans involving other agencies.

The generalist confronting someone with a severe ED—especially anorexia nervosa (AN)—may be uncertain as to whom the patient is best referred. The worried family or friends may insist that 'something must be done'. The clinician may agree but the question of what should be done and by whom is not always straightforward.

Box 10.1 National Service Framework

'Individuals with severe eating disorders should be referred for specialist assessment including a full medical and psychiatric assessment'.

ABC of Eating Disorders. Edited by J. Morris. © 2008 Blackwell Publishing, ISBN: 978-0-7279-1843-7.

Physical emergency

For a small minority of cases, the clinician may consider that the patient is in immediate danger. The patient may collapse, feel very unwell or have some severe biochemical abnormality such as a potassium level of 2.1 mmol/L. If the GP judges that admission or at least hospital assessment is necessary, then urgent referral to the local general medical service is indicated. Most physicians receiving the referral will not have any particular or special expertise in EDs, but s/he should be able to further assess and stabilize the patient's physical state. However, most admissions onto medical wards for physical 'rescue' are brief and leave unresolved the question of who is to try to treat the ED itself. The GP needs to make a parallel referral to some 'specialist' who will undertake this task. But who should it be?

Who treats people with eating disorders?

The answer is an array of people mainly within mental health services. Furthermore, the answer will be different in different places. Until the last decade or so, few places had specialist services in the sense of services dedicated solely to the treatment of EDs. This is still the case in many places and is usual with child and adolescent mental health services (CAMHS) where the treatment of EDs is commonly construed as part of the core business of generalist teams. In these cases, the initial referral would be to the general mental health services, often to the relevant community mental health team (CMHT). Furthermore, even when there is a local specialist ED team it may be defined as a 'tertiary' service accepting referrals only via general mental health teams.

What if there is no local specialist service?

In those areas of the country where no specialist ED service is available, patients with EDs are usually managed by generic adult mental health teams. The degree of competence and confidence about treating EDs available within generalist CMHTs varies widely. Thus with luck the relevant team may include one or two professionals who have special interest in working with ED patients. However, some CMHTs argue that they lack the skills to manage ED patients or that such patients fall outside their remit of managing severe mental illness. If the CMHT takes such a position, the trust of which they form a part and/or the primary care trust that has the remit to organize services should be quizzed directly as to what provision has been made for people with EDs. If necessary they should be reminded that EDs are mental disorders and are often as severe as psychoses in terms of both morbidity and mortality and also burden to carers. If there is no local service, there may well agreements with neighbouring services or with voluntary or private provisions but these rarely add up to a satisfactorily comprehensive response to the whole range of EDs. The NICE guideline sets out the interventions that are reasonable but not how they are best organized (Figure 10.1).

Specialist services, what are they?

The present trend is toward the development of specialist local teams and services for the management of EDs in adults (Figures 10.2 & 10.3). However, in general such development has been uncoordinated and piecemeal. A bit of history may be helpful. Over most of the last 50 years or so, the only specialist services for

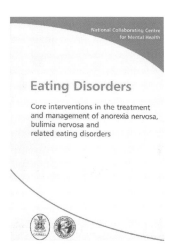

Figure 10.1 The National Institute for Clinical Excellence Guideline *Eating Disorders*. (NICE 2004)

EDs in the UK were those initiated by a small number of interested psychiatrists and a few physicians, mainly in academic centres. As a result, such services developed in an uneven way and tended to emphasize the inpatient treatment of AN. In response to this patchiness, private inpatient units grew in numbers in the 1990s when new arrangements simplified the funding of the private treatment of National Health Service (NHS) patients. However, recently more special NHS services have been and are being created. Thus, in 2000 a survey by the Eating Disorders Special Interest Group of the Royal College of Psychiatrists found that specialist services for adults had increased in number from 21 in 1991 to 39 in 2000. There have been more created since the second report. Nevertheless, many areas of the country remain without access to nearby specialist services.

Services or teams who may be called 'specialist' should have available appropriate clinicians who are able to assess, monitor and treat patients with EDs. Assessment needs to be multidimensional, involving the psychological, the social and physical. Teams consist of people with different skills. Clinicians working in those services may be drawn from a variety of professions such as medicine, nursing, dietetics, clinical psychology and occupational therapy. With appropriate training and support, together with a measure of flexibility, any or all of these clinicians may undertake the role of therapist and case managers. However, if the team does not have medical members, the issue of how the physical issues and risks are to be managed poses important questions that cannot be ignored although they may be answered in more ways than one. A similar although perhaps less clear-cut question concerns the management of major psychiatric comorbidity.

Types of specialist service

Specialist services come in different shapes and forms. Some of them are primarily outpatient based. Others also offer inpatient treatment and/or a day treatment facility. A few are pioneering intensive domiciliary care. Some accept referrals of people with any kind of ED whilst others may accept only people with AN or complex and difficult cases. Some focus upon supervising and supporting their generalist

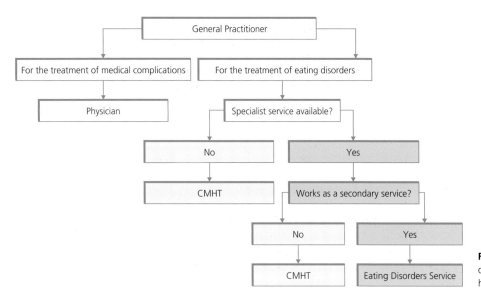

Figure 10.2 Referring adults with eating disorders. CMHT, community mental health team.

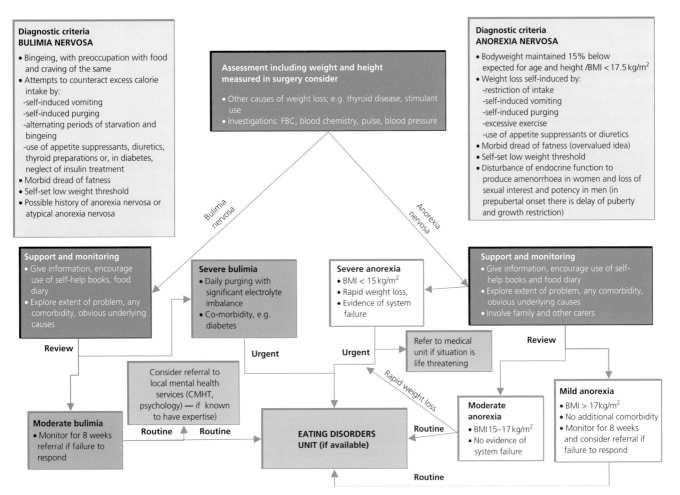

Figure 10.3 Primary care protocol for the management of adults with eating disorders. BMI, body mass index; CMHT, community mental health team; FBC, full blood count. (Royal College of Psychiatrists 2000)

Box 10.2 **What a comprehensive service for anorexia nervosa should provide**

- Assessment—psychosocial and physical
- Potentially long-term therapy
- Availability of more intensive care
- Management of psychiatric comorbidity
- Management of physical complications
- Involvement of families and others as appropriate
- Follow-up and good communication

Box 10.3 **What a comprehensive service for bulimia nervosa should provide**

- Assessment—psychosocial and physical
- Effective short-term psychotherapy
- Other therapies—'self-help' drugs, psycho-education
- Follow-up and additional therapy for those who do not respond
- Special or prolonged therapy for complicated cases
- Management of psychiatric comorbidity
- Management of physical complications
- Follow-up and good communication

colleagues. Some exclude people with binge eating disorder (BED) or even all forms of atypical disorder or eating disorder not otherwise stated (EDNOS) even though evidence suggests that such cases are common and of a similar severity to more 'typical' disorders.

Thus many services fall well short of being 'comprehensive' in the sense of being able to offer the full range of interventions set out on Boxes 10.2 and 10.3. Services that have major limitations need to be honest about what they can and cannot provide and they should also be able to assist referring clinicians in facilitating access to other services.

What happens if the local eating disorder service does not include inpatient treatment and the patient requires admission?

The commonest way that an ED service may fall short of being comprehensive is that it does not have an inpatient facility. This is especially relevant for people with severe AN.

Most people with AN should be managed on an outpatient basis with psychological treatment provided by a service that is competent in giving that treatment and assessing the physical risk of people with EDs. However, a minority of patients do require inpatient treatment and in the absence of suitable beds locally arranging this may involve jumping a number of hurdles not least being the securing of funding.

When a patient with severe AN does need admission it should be to a unit that can provide the skilled implementation of refeeding with careful physical monitoring in combination with psychosocial interventions. Ideally, this should be provided within reasonable travelling distance so as to enable the involvement of relatives and carers in treatment and the maintenance of social and occupational links. However this is not always possible.

When patients are admitted to distant units, the local ED service—or if there is none the local generic service—together with the GP should remain in close touch during the admission and be involved in timely planning of an ongoing care plan. Such coordination is easier if the local service and the tertiary unit have established links over time and more difficult when the arrangement is a one off.

What happens to children?

Children and adolescents who develop EDs whilst they are under 16 years of age (under 18 years in some cases) or still at school are usually managed by the local CAMHS (Figure 10.4). Specialist outpatient EDs services for children and adolescents are rare in the UK. The need for inpatient treatment for urgent weight restoration should be balanced alongside the educational and social needs of the young person. However, when children and adolescents do require inpatient care, admission should be to an age-appropriate setting. This may be to a paediatric bed, to a generic adolescent unit, or to a specialized inpatient facility often in the private sector.

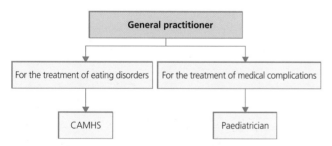

Figure 10.4 Referring children and adolescents with eating disorders. CAMHS, child and adolescent mental health services.

(Children below 12 years of age are usually managed in paediatric beds as there are very few specialist EDs beds for them.) Nearly a quarter of all beds in CAMHS inpatient units in England and Wales are occupied by patients with EDs.

Transitions

Eating disorders are commonly long lasting. Many young people eventually need to be transferred from CAMHS to adult services. The move is often complicated as there may be a sudden change in treatment ethos towards increased individual responsibility which may feel bewildering and dangerous for patients and their families. Parents may feel excluded from decisions about care. Successful transitions from CAMHS to adult services are more likely when the relevant patients are identified in good time and the adult ED team becomes involved in their care well before the transfer.

The treatment of students in higher education may involve another challenging transition. The move to and from university and home may complicate the delivery of psychological treatments and make the involvement of family in therapy impractical.

Few services are designed to accommodate such problems and an increased burden may fall upon University Counselling Services which may or may not be able to provide what is necessary.

Further reading

Arcelus J & Button E. Clinical and socio-demographic characteristics of university students referred to an eating disorders service. *European Eating Disorders Review* 2007; **15**: 146–151.

Gowers SG, Weetman J, Shore A *et al*. Impact of hospitalization on the outcome of adolescent anorexia nervosa. *British Journal of Psychiatry* 2000; **176**: 138–141.

NICE. *Eating Disorders: Core Interventions in the Treatment and Management of Anorexia Nervosa, Bulimia Nervosa and Related Eating Disorders.* NICE Clinical Guideline No 9. National Institute for Clinical Excellence, London, 2004: http://www.nice.org.uk

Royal College of Psychiatrists. *Eating Disorders in the UK: Policies for Service Development and Training. Council Report CR87.* Royal College of Psychiatrists, London, 2000.

Royal College of Psychiatrists. *The Mental Health of Students in Higher Education (Council report CRI12).* Royal College of Psychiatrists, London, 2003.

Treasure J, Schmidt U & Hugo P. Mind the gap: service transition and interface problems for patients with eating disorders. *British Journal of Psychiatry* 2005; **187**: 398–400.

CHAPTER 11

Medico-legal and Ethical Issues in the Treatment of Eating Disorders

Anne Stewart and Jacinta Tan

OVERVIEW

- Ethical and legal issues often arise in the management of eating disorders and require careful consideration by the clinician.

- Assessment of the right to refuse treatment involves assessing how risky the condition is, what the likely benefit or harm of treatment is, whether the patient is competent to make a reasoned choice and whether the patients and/or family can engage in other treatment options.

- Healthy decision-making should be promoted, by providing information on what is entailed in treatment and the risks and benefits of having or not having treatment, by building up a treatment alliance and by taking a collaborative and motivational approach.

- Legal routes to compulsory care include the use of the Mental Health Act (MHA), the Mental Capacity Act (MCA) or in the case of minors, parental consent or Child Care Law.

- With minors, it is important to listen to the young person's views. However, parents or other adults may have the right to require the young person to have treatment, even if they appear competent to refuse treatment.

- Confidentiality should be respected as far as possible but may need to be overridden in order to prevent serious harm to the patient.

Box 11.1 **Some ethical principles that can be applied to the treatment of eating disorders: Beauchamp and Childress' Four Principles**

Beneficence
- Taking an approach that ensures that the treatments offered are likely to be beneficial.

Non-maleficence
- Taking an approach that minimizes the harmful effects of treatment.

Autonomy
- Promoting the autonomy of patients wherever possible.

Justice
- Ensuring that patients have a fair and equitable access to treatment.
- Ensuring protection of human rights e.g. to fair treatment, confidentiality, protection of dignity.

Introduction

Ethical and legal issues often arise in the management of eating disorders and need careful consideration by clinicians (Box 11.1). A particular problem is the reluctance of some patients to accept treatment or even acknowledge that they have a problem, despite suffering serious physical, psychological or social consequences of the disorder. For young people, the eating disorder may have become a way of asserting themselves or gaining control within their family; giving up the eating disorder means giving up that control (Figure 11.1). Refusal of treatment is common both in adults and young people and can pose a difficult dilemma for the clinician. The consequences of not giving treatment may be life threatening,

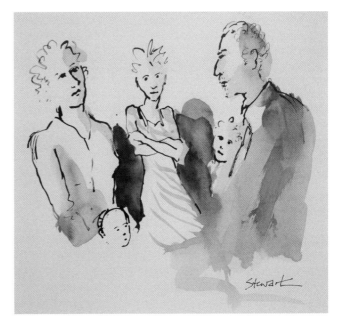

Figure 11.1 Taking control in the family. (Drawing by kind permission of Robin Stewart)

ABC of Eating Disorders. Edited by J. Morris. © 2008 Blackwell Publishing, ISBN: 978-0-7279-1843-7.

Box 11.2 **Case vignette: Alison**

Alison is a young adult who lives at home with her parents. She started dieting at 16 years of age following stresses in her family and the break-up of a relationship with a boyfriend. She became very preoccupied with her body image and began to lose weight. Her parents tried to encourage her to eat but were concerned about the conflict that ensued. Alison became very secretive and did not keep her parents informed about her weight loss and physical state. Although very low in weight, she managed to start a university course. However, in her second year she was sent home due to further loss of weight and her deteriorating physical condition. She maintains that there is nothing wrong with her and that she needs to be left alone to get on with her life. When questioned she says that she is too fat and needs to lose more weight. Her parents discover her one day having fainted and call their family doctor. Her pulse rate is 45, blood pressure is low and body mass index (BMI) is 14. She refuses to come into hospital and does not want her parents to know the result of her assessment. Her parents are at a loss as to how to help her.

Box 11.3 **Determining the right to refuse treatment: factors to take into account**

- How risky is their current condition?
- What is the likely benefit and harm of treatment?
- Is the patient competent to make a reasoned choice?
- Can the patient and/or family engage in other treatment options?

yet the clinician may wish to respect the autonomy of the patient in order to maintain a therapeutic relationship. With patients who are legal minors, the necessity for parental involvement can add to the complexity of management.

Another key ethical and legal dilemma relates to confidentiality. This is particularly pertinent to young people and adults who are living at home but reluctant to disclose details of their disorder to family members.

These dilemmas are highlighted in the case vignette (Box 11.2).

Determination of the right to refuse treatment

Like Alison in the case vignette (see Box 11.2), many people with eating disorders insist that they do not wish to have treatment. There are a number of factors which need to be taken into account in order to determine whether this refusal should be respected (Box 11.3).

How risky is their current condition?

A thorough assessment is needed in order to determine the medical and psychiatric risk (see Box 11.4 for a summary of serious physical consequences). Rapid weight loss can increase the risk, alongside the risk relating to low weight. An assessment of the presence of severe depression or suicidal thoughts is also crucial as part of the risk assessment; eating disorders carry the highest mortality of

Box 11.4 **Factors indicating high risk**

Physical factors
- Low weight
- Rapid weight loss whether or not there is low weight
- Low blood pressure/pulse
- Chest pain
- Reduced exercise tolerance
- Renal dysfunction or low urine output
- Muscle weakness
- Disturbed blood indices (particularly low haemoglobin and white cell count, low sodium or potassium levels, raised urea, abnormal liver function

Psychiatric factors
- Severe depression
- Suicidal behaviour

any of the functional psychiatric disorders (deaths result from both medical causes and suicide).

What is the likely benefit and harm of treatment?

In considering whether to impose treatment, it is important to weigh up carefully the potential benefits of treatment against the possible harmful effects. Evidence-based treatments should be offered wherever possible.

In the UK the National Institute for Health and Clinical Excellence (NICE) guidelines (NICE 2004) provide an appraisal of the best evidence available regarding the management of anorexia nervosa, bulimia nervosa and related disorders in individuals aged 8 years and over. Key recommendations based on evidence include the use of cognitive behavioural therapy in the treatment of bulimia nervosa in adults and the involvement of families in treatments that directly address the eating disorder in young people. The NICE guidelines specify that outpatient treatment should be tried first wherever possible.

The evidence base regarding inpatient treatment is lacking, with no controlled trials. Those treated compulsorily may have a poorer outcome than those treated voluntarily. However, it is difficult to tease out the effect of severity. An outcome study of young people with eating disorders found poorer outcome with respect to social, psychological and family functioning in those admitted for inpatient treatment. Thus, although both inpatient admission and treatment under compulsion may be life saving, the possible adverse effects also need to be considered.

As well as the general factors just considered, it is important to weigh up, with the individual patient, the effect of inpatient or compulsory treatment on motivation, collaboration and morale. An inpatient admission may achieve the goal of weight gain, but, if collaboration has not been achieved, weight may be lost following discharge. It is possible, however, to achieve collaboration within the framework of inpatient treatment, even if the admission is compulsory. Recent research indicates that what is most important for patients is whether they are respected and listened to, rather than whether the treatment is compulsory or voluntary.

Box 11.5 **Criteria for determining capacity in England and Wales (From The Mental Capacity Act 2005)**

A person is unable to make a decision for himself if he is unable:
(a) to understand the information relevant to the decision;
(b) to retain that information;
(c) to use or weigh that information as part of the process of making the decision; or
(d) to communicate his decision (whether by talking, using sign language or any other means).

Is the patient competent to make a reasoned choice?

In order to determine whether a patient should have the right to refuse treatment it is important to assess whether they have the capacity to make this decision. The legal criteria for determining capacity may differ slightly between countries. The criteria for England and Wales are detailed in Box 11.5.

Some patients with eating disorders may appear to have capacity yet their decision-making may still be adversely affected by their illness. Research has shown that having an eating disorder can impact on the patient's sense of identity and values, thus impairing the ability to make decisions from a broader perspective, even if intellectual capacity is retained. In assessing competence it is important to take into account previous values, personality and identity of the patient.

Can the patient and/or family engage in other treatment options?

It is important to ascertain whether the patient is willing and able to engage in other treatment options. In the case of young people it is important to explore in detail how the parents will be able to keep the young person safe at home and promote recovery.

How to promote good decision-making

There are a number of strategies that help to promote healthy decision-making, shown in Box 11.6. As long as the patient is not at serious risk it may be appropriate to take time to build up a treatment alliance and ensure that decision-making is collaborative as far as is possible. Taking a motivational approach can enable the patient to consider for themselves the pros and cons of treatment, their goals and the impact of the eating disorder on their goals. Ideally, they are then in a better position to make a decision which is right for them.

Legal routes to compulsory treatment (Box 11.7)

Despite the best attempts to work collaboratively, a patient may continue to refuse treatment. If the risks are serious, and inpatient treatment is in the best interest of the patient, compulsory treatment may be necessary.

Each country has different laws governing the use of treatment without the patient's consent. There can be more than one possible

Box 11.6 **How to promote competent decision-making**

- Provide information about the eating disorder and its consequences.
- Provide information on what is entailed in treatment.
- Take time to go through the risks and benefits of treatment and of not having treatment.
- Provide a setting which is free of distractions or interruptions.
- Take time to build up a treatment alliance.
- Ensure that decision-making is collaborative, as far as is possible.
- Take a motivational approach.
- Clarify the advantages and disadvantages from the patient's point of view of having an eating disorder.
- Enable the patient to consider for themselves the pros and cons of treatment.
- Help patients to consider their short-term and long-term goals.
- Help patients to consider the impact of the eating disorder on their goals.
- Encourage patient to make a decision that is right for them.

Box 11.7 **Routes to compulsory treatment**

- Mental health legislation for the protection and treatment of those with mental disorders.
- Mental incapacity law or guardianship law for the protection of those who lack capacity to make their own decisions.
- Law governing emergency and life-saving treatment if required before full assessments can be done or legal measures instituted.
- Child care law (for those who are legal minors) governing the protection and welfare of young people.
- Parental consent laws (for legal minors).

legal route to such compulsory treatment, including invoking laws concerning treatment of mental illnesses, overriding treatment refusal in cases of mental incapacity and appointing guardians for vulnerable patients.

Issues to consider with young people

For legal minors, there are additional considerations such as the protection of children and ensuring their continued welfare and development. Legally, parents or others may have the right to require minors to receive treatment in their best interests even if they are competent to refuse it. Clearly, it is important to listen to the young person's views throughout and respect their wishes as far as possible. At the same time, factors such as the level of maturity and independence of the young person should be considered, so that they can be enabled to make as many decisions as possible and participate in all decision-making, without burdening them with inappropriate responsibilities. It may become necessary in certain circumstances for parents and professionals to take charge to ensure that the young person receive the necessary treatment in order to recover from their eating disorder. This can generally be done under parental consent. As they gradually improve and become more mature and able to take charge of themselves, it is important to continue to build collaboration and encourage increasing autonomy and choice. With older adolescents, or where there is persistent resistance to receiving inpatient treatment, the use of formal legal means may be more appropriate than parental consent.

There may be circumstances where parents are unwilling for their young person to have treatment, even though the young person is seriously ill. In this case, it may be necessary to consider whether the parents are acting in the best interests of their child, and invoke child care law to ensure that the child receives appropriate care.

An ethical decision-making framework (Figure 11.2)

Figure 11.2 shows a framework for managing a patient who is refusing treatment. The first step is to engage the patient and seek to understand the context and the reasons for treatment refusal. It is essential to carry out a comprehensive assessment in order to determine the physical and psychiatric risks. The second step is to provide information regarding their disorder and its consequences, and to discuss carefully the treatment options, including the risks and benefits of treatment. It is important, if possible, to give time to explore and manage any anxieties or concerns, in order to arrive at joint decision-making. Families should be involved wherever possible. Where there is reluctance to accept treatment it is important to explore the reasons for this. Throughout this process it is important to promote a sense of autonomy in the patient, whilst, at the same time, providing the necessary support and boundaries.

If it is not possible to agree on treatment, then there needs to be a consideration of the risks involved. If the risks are such

that an admission is advisable but not essential, then another safe option can be agreed and further time taken to build trust. If admission is considered to be essential, then the decision to admit compulsorily under mental health act legislation may need to be taken.

If the patient requires compulsory admission then it is important to ensure that treatment is experienced as supportive and facilitative, rather than coercive or punitive. It is helpful to view treatment refusal as being part of an evolving collaborative process.

A cornerstone of ethical practice is good team work. Relationships between team members can become difficult particularly if there are high risks involved; differences of opinion may mirror splits within the family. Developing a respectful and collaborative way of working within teams can facilitate effective and efficient clinical work.

Consideration of confidentiality and fair access to treatment

Many young people who are still legal minors do not wish their parents to know the details of their disorder and treatment. The right to confidentiality is built on the assumption that patients are able to take reasoned decisions about sharing information with others. Professionals (and parents) need to promote this skill in young people. However, information may need to be shared against the wishes of the young person where it is in their best interest and the young person needs care and protection. It is important to enable the young person to exercise their right to confidentiality in other ways, for example: allowing them to keep private the details of their individual therapy.

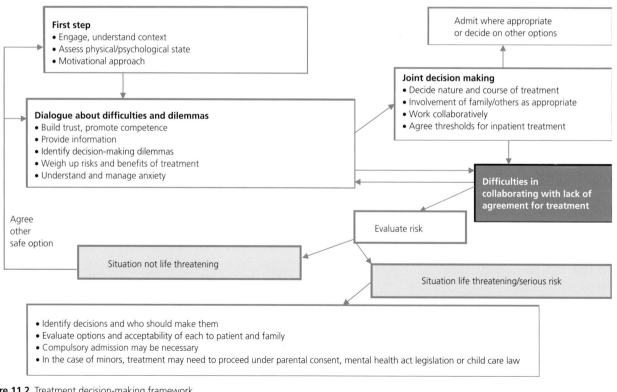

Figure 11.2 Treatment decision-making framework.

A young adult with an eating disorder living with his or her parents and adults living with partners or spouses may be unwilling to disclose details of their progress and treatment. In general, it is helpful to include parents and carers within treatment reviews in order that the most appropriate support is given. Wherever possible, permission should be obtained from the patient for sharing information with carers. If confidentiality has to be breached, to prevent serious harm to the patient, it should be done in a manner which is respectful and caring.

Confidentiality within health care teams is also a pertinent issue, with the growing computerization of records and ease of transfer of information. Health care teams have an obligation to keep their records safe and to be clear with the patient who has access to information. In order for teams to work safely together there must be sharing of information. However, it is important to consider carefully who needs to know any specific information. Communication with schools or social services may go beyond the boundaries of medical confidentiality and is therefore usually undertaken only with consent from the patient and with clear aims. An exception to this is where there are child protection concerns, when it is crucial to contact social services.

Finally, a further ethical consideration is ensuring that patients have fair access to appropriate treatment. Minimizing inequities in treatment and striving to improve treatments through research, evaluation, audit and training is an important aspect of an ethical approach.

Summary

Eating disorders, by their nature, can be particularly ethically and legally challenging. Health professionals should consider the ethical and legal issues involved as they evaluate the physical and psychological needs of patients. Where compulsory treatment needs to be undertaken, the legal and ethical principles should be explicit to the patient and the treatment carried out sensitively and respectfully in order to maximize collaboration.

Further reading

Goldner EM, Birmingham CL & Smye V. Addressing treatment refusal in anorexia nervosa. Clinical, ethical and legal considerations. In: Garner DM & Garfinkel PE, eds. *Handbook of Treatment for Eating Disorders*, 2nd edn. Guilford Press, New York, 1997: 450–461.

Gowers SG, Weetman J, Shore A *et al*. Impact of hospitalisation on the outcome of adolescent anorexia nervosa. *British Journal of Psychiatry* 2000; **176**: 138–141.

NICE. *Eating Disorders: Core Interventions in the Treatment and Management of Anorexia Nervosa, Bulimia Nervosa and Related Eating Disorders*. NICE Clinical Guideline No 9. National Institute for Clinical Excellence, London, 2004: http://www.nice.org.uk

Rathner G. A plea against compulsory treatment of anorexia nervosa. In: Vanderycken W & Beaumont PJ, eds. *Treating Eating Disorders: Ethical, Legal and Personal Issues*. Athlone Press, London, 1998: 179–215.

Stewart A & Tan J. Ethical and legal issues. In: Lask B & Bryant-Waugh R, eds. *Eating Disorders in Childhood and Early Adolescence*, 3rd edn. Guilford Press, New York, 2007: 335–359.

Tan JOA, Hope T & Stewart A. Anorexia nervosa and personal identity: the accounts of patients and their parents. *International Journal of Law and Psychiatry* 2003; **26**: 533–548.

Tan JOA, Hope T, Stewart A & Fitzpatrick R. Competence to refuse treatment in anorexia nervosa. *International Journal of Law and Psychiatry* 2003; **26**: 697–707.

Tan JOA, Hope T, Stewart A & Fitzpatrick R. Control and compulsory treatment in anorexia nervosa: the views of patients and parents. *International Journal of Law and Psychiatry* 2003; **26**(6): 627–645.

Tan JOA, Stewart A, Fitzpatrick R & Hope T. Competence to make treatment decisions in anorexia nervosa: thinking processes and values. *Philosophy, Psychology and Psychiatry* 2006; **13**: 267–282.

Vanderycken W & Beaumont PJ, eds. *Treating Eating Disorders: Ethical, Legal and Personal Issues*. Athlone Press, London, 1998.

CHAPTER 12

Children with Eating and Feeding Disorders

Jane Morris and Fiona Forbes

Epidemiology of eating disorders in children

Both extremes of weight are problems for young people today—among adolescents the three most common chronic medical conditions are obesity, asthma and anorexia nervosa (AN). More child and adolescent psychiatric beds are occupied by young people with AN than any other group.

Ninety per cent of sufferers of postpubertal eating disorders are female. Among children and young teenagers, though, sex ratios are more even. Unhealthily low weight is harder to detect in children, since it may take the form of failure to *gain* weight and height. Body mass index (BMI) alone may appear normal. Furthermore, normal BMI range is lower in younger children, so that a BMI diagnostic of AN in an 18-year-old girl can be perfectly healthy for a 12-year-old boy.

This underscores the value of cumulative growth charts for children (Figure 12.1a,b). Health visitors' records may be supplemented by school records, and predicted height may be calculated from the parental heights. British schools would benefit from the Scandinavian system where pupils are weighed and measured

ABC of Eating Disorders. Edited by J. Morris. © 2008 Blackwell Publishing, ISBN: 978-0-7279-1843-7.

annually, allowing early intervention and advice for underweight or overweight children.

Eating and feeding disorders in children are more likely to present atypically (Boxes 12.1 & 12.2). Weight loss is not an invariable feature, and overvaluation of bodily weight and shape may be absent too. Food may be shunned for reasons other than its 'fattening' capacity. There may be phobia of choking or being sick. Conversely, children described as 'failing to thrive' (weight below the third centile or showing progressive weight loss), may not suffer from psychological difficulties in eating but from their parents' inability to provide adequate nourishment for whatever reason.

How do eating disorders present before puberty?

Although children are more likely than adults to present with 'feeding disorders', cases of classic AN or bulimia nervosa (BN), are increasingly reported in prepubertal children. In retrospect, many patients with AN and BN first developed symptoms in childhood or early adolescence, but they rarely receive treatment until the mid-teens, or even adulthood, particularly in the case of BN where weight remains normal. This may mean the loss of a window of opportunity for early intervention. On the other hand, some of these disorders may be transient and resolve spontaneously.

The distinction between eating disorders and other feeding disorders: what's different, what's the same? (Box 12.2)

The younger the child, the more urgent it becomes to investigate physical causes of malnutrition, and social and traumatic aetiologies for failure to thrive. Physical, emotional and sexual abuse certainly do not lie behind all cases, and where abuse is investigated and managed, care must be taken to refeed a malnourished child if s/he is to participate healthily in therapy and catch up on normal development.

Eating and feeding disorders of the very young need multidisciplinary evaluation involving physical investigations from developmental paediatrician, dietician (food diaries), growth charts and psychiatric assessment. Family history and involvement are crucial, and it is illuminating to observe a family meal, preferably in the home.

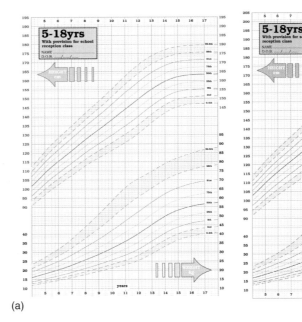

Figure 12.1 Growth charts for (a) girls and (b) boys. © Child Growth Foundation.

(a)

(b)

Box 12.1 Case vignette: Jon—food avoidant emotional disorder (FAED)

Jon, a small, timid 12-year-old boy, had an episode of 'food poisoning' and developed a great fear of being sick. He avoided more and more different foods which he considered put him at risk, insisted on obsessive hygiene around food, and began to avoid journeys in case of travel sickness or being offered food in a strange place. He would not eat at all in school.

He lost weight precipitously. Starvation intensified his obsessive symptoms—he would only eat from certain dishes, which all had to be washed in a ritualistic way. His mother, a part-time secretary, was 'at her wits end'—she had never known Jon to have tantrums like those he now threw if she tried to make him eat. She went along with his wishes until his younger sister protested to grandparents and the family sought treatment.

Jonathan was diagnosed with FAED. Diagnoses of both Asberger's syndrome and obsessive compulsive disorder were considered. Obsessionality is made very much worse by starvation—a vicious circle can develop. Treatment **must** include refeeding, and Jon was also offered cognitive-behavioural sessions, backed up by parallel family work and selective serotonin reuptake inhibitors (SSRIs), such as Sertraline, in anticompulsive doses.

Jonathon accepted a regime of supplement drinks which improved his weight and psychological state somewhat, but refused to take any medication when he discovered nausea was a possible side-effect.

Luckily, his obsessive symptoms responded well to weight gain and behavioural treatment with intensive family support. He grew 6 inches in height in as many months and remained slim but no longer emaciated as he now ate enough to keep pace with the enormous demands of puberty. He was delighted by the growth spurt and by his increased muscle bulk. There was a brief setback when he first returned to school. He became clingy and tearful and the family considered moving him to a small private school. Jon insisted that he wanted to stay among his friends, however, and managed to persevere.

Box 12.2 Eating disorders versus other eating/feeding disorders: what's different, what's the same?

What's the same?
- Physical risks of starvation if there is weight loss.
- Need to normalize physical state in order to address psychological issues fruitfully.
- Avoidance likely to be a prominent feature.
- Severe obsessional symptoms likely.
- May be a family history of eating or feeding disorder, and unusual mealtime behaviour in the family.
- Whatever the origins of the disorder, 'secondary gain' very likely in children.
- Family need tactful support to change behaviour to avoid reinforcing pathology.
- Extreme anxiety when habitual ritualistic practices or avoidance challenged.
- Shame and secrecy likely to be an issue in both sufferer and family.

What's different?
- In anorexia nervosa and bulimia nervosa the core feature is overevaluation of body weight and shape, and the drive is for thinness.
- Not only starvation/food avoidance but overexercise/purging/ courting cold/use of slimming remedies to lose calories—all dangerous to health.
- Patients with anorexia nervosa more likely to resist all attempts at refeeding (including tube-feeding) than in other disorders.

The key distinguishing feature of AN and BN is the undue overe-valuation of body weight and shape. Cultural attitudes towards body shape are felt at school and even nursery. Children and young people with AN or BN will show preferences for low calorie, low fat or 'diet' foods—but very young patients may harbour misconceptions

328-1-58 No 7430 3 JANUARY 2004 *Clinical research* ISSN 0959-8138

Box 12.3 **Checklist of feeding/eating disorders in children**

- Failure to thrive (*physical or social causes*)
- Selective eating (*extreme faddiness*)
- Restrictive eating (*child has small appetite and eats normal range of food but in small amounts*)
- Functional dysphagia (*fear of choking or vomiting—certain foods avoided*)
- Food refusal (*act of refusal rather than search for thinness*)
- Pervasive refusal disorder (*may be a consequence of severe trauma*)
- Food avoidance emotional disorder (FAED) (*mood disturbance with weight loss*)
- Obsessive compulsive disorder (OCD) (*with eating rituals and other rituals*)
- Weight loss associated with psychostimulants
- Anorexia and bulimia nervosa in younger children

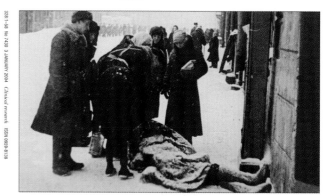

3 January 2004

BMJ

Leningrad: the long term effects of starvation

Starvation in puberty may lead to later cardiovascular disease p11

Antidepressants in children p3
Does a stable partnership protect against progression to AIDS? p15
Radiation to the brain during infancy damages cognition p19
Reinventing academic medicine p43
Time to ditch the white coat? p57

bmj.com

Figure 12.2 Cover of *BMJ*, vol. 328, 3 January 2004, with kind permission of *BMJ*.

about nutritional values and 'magical' beliefs, such as the notion that calories can 'infect' the body by touch or smell alone. They will probably engage in other weight loss behaviours, such as overexercising or wearing few clothes to 'shiver away' calories.

An underweight child who appears to have psychotic or obsessive-compulsive symptoms should not be 'labelled' until after a trial of weight gain—many symptoms vanish or at least mitigate with adequate nutrition. The 'antidepressant' effects of food are also very gratifying to observe in a refed child.

Children with feeding disorders often appear 'stuck' with extreme forms of behaviour more characteristic of earlier stages of development. The developmental perspective is crucial—the 'faddiness' normal in a 2-year-old child is socially and psychologically abnormal in a 12-year-old child. 'Selective eating' is a common transient problem in most toddlers, 'food refusal' is common in tiny children, and some children take longer than expected to be weaned from sloppy foods to solids. When such delays become chronic and extreme, and particularly if other symptoms are added (children with food refusal may also refuse to wash, attend school or even to speak), families or other concerned agencies seek help. Feeding disorders may be associated with emaciation, overweight or normal weight, although they are more likely to present if weight falls.

Behavioural restoration of healthy weight and healthy eating behaviour is important but not always sufficient. Any trauma, neglect or difficult interpersonal issues must be solved if a child is to respond in a lasting way. Sometimes eating problems reflect physical illness or its treatment (cystic fibrosis, diabetes, steroid treatment) or result from psychiatric disorders (autistic spectrum, obsessive compulsive disorder, psychoses) which must be addressed in parallel with the refeeding efforts.

Medication can reduce appetite. Children on methylphenidate for attention deficit hyperactivity disorder (ADHD) should have their growth monitored and charted. Thoughtful prescribing allows concentration and calm by day, with a rest from medication in the evening, when the child eats the main meal. Try to omit medication at weekends and school holidays if the family can cope.

Other medications cause appetite gain. It is unrealistic and unkind to expect young people to exert 'will-power' without considerable help, particularly when their psychiatric condition already makes demands on the young mind. Wherever possible prescribers should consider 'appetite-neutral' alternatives—quetiapine rather than olanzapine, for instance, for young women with psychosis.

Particular physical, psychological and social risks for children with eating and feeding disorders

There is particular urgency about refeeding underweight children. The smaller the child the faster the dehydration and deterioration. Paediatric metabolism is faster than adults' and physical growth and exposure to new infection add further demands. Starvation at times of crucial physiological growth may cause long-term damage. Starvation in 10–14 year olds during the Siege of Leningrad (Figure 12.2) was associated with higher blood pressure, cholesterol levels and overall mortality in the survivors half a century later, and studies of the Dutch Famine of 1944 have yielded similar findings, as well as insights into second generation consequences of starvation in pregnant women.

Skeletal growth too may be retarded, with permanent stunting of height in those starved during puberty. We do not yet know the effects of malnutrition on a still-developing brain. The frontal lobe develops strikingly during adolescence, with both profusion and pruning of neural connexions (Giedd *et al.*), reflected in growing social maturity and capacity for abstract thought, but patients with severe AN continue to function in a concrete, childlike way despite academic success and superficial 'grown-upness'.

Cognitive function is impaired by short-term starvation, and by vomiting—with enormous individual variation. Considerable recovery occurs with renutrition, allowing better engagement in psychological therapies. Social and psychological development is seriously compromised by illness, particularly by hospitalization. Luckily, the presence of a 'good enough' family can often substitute for inpatient care, and it is acceptable for parents to take physical charge of feeding young children when necessary. (The role of the family is considered in more detail in Chapter 13.)

Orchestration of a coordinated systemic response—involving at least family, school and medical professionals—is a complicated task, not to be underestimated. Clinicians should expect the child to instinctively behave in a way which protects anorexic behaviour and brings about maximum confusion and disruption to the therapeutic process. School is a particularly difficult arena—return to school is often not a sign of health and progress but a retreat from adult supervision where anorexic behaviours flourish.

Management of eating disorders in children: what's different, what's the same?

Refeeding any starved patient is essential to allow effective psychological input. This must be done calmly and with understanding of the underlying difficulty, since high arousal and aggressive coercion build a vicious cycle.

The importance of diagnosing AN or BN is that addressing the disordered eating and weight will not bring about lasting improvement unless educational and motivational work are undertaken as soon as the child's cognitive function allows this. When a feeding disorder has a different aetiology, the root psychopathology must be addressed in its own right. Sometimes a period of starvation and disordered eating from other causes can act as a trigger for AN itself in a predisposed individual. Our culture values slimness to a pathological extent, and 'fat' is the most shaming of playground insults. The two types of disorder can become enmeshed and are not mutually exclusive.

Prescription of antidepressant drugs for children is controversial and certainly unlikely to be effective at low weight. High antiobsessional doses of selective serotonin reuptake inhibitors (SSRIs) can exert useful effects on obsessive-compulsive symptoms, however, if these persist despite weight gain. The use of olanzapine in facilitating feeding at low weight is best left to hospital specialists.

There is no 'quick fix' for AN, and it cannot be assumed that any intelligent child who is shown the physical dangers of starvation will be frightened into eating normally again. Indeed the child's indifference in contrast with parents' increasing fearful concern may widen the gulf between them. The best approach is to gradually and repeatedly make the links between the symptoms the child dislikes—weariness, agitation, sleep problems, feeling the cold, loss of friendships, inability to join in socially, falling sport or academic performance, 'fussing' by parents—and the anorexia. It is then useful to help the child notice how weight gain brings the corresponding benefits—more energy, calm, resistance to cold, growing in height (it is generally 'cool' to be tall), capacity to have fun with friends and being well enough to join in games again.

We should acknowledge sympathetically—not angrily—the benefits which undoubtedly come with a serious eating disorder: its power to oblige people to care and placate, the relief from social and sexual demands, the sense that one's body is now controlled rather than terrifyingly unpredictable. Young patients need new techniques for coping with these aspects of life without having to starve.

Further reading

Douglas J. Psychological treatment of food refusal in young children. *Child & Adolescent Mental Health* 2002; **7**(4): 173–180.

Fox C & Joughin C. *Childhood Onset Eating Problems: Findings from Research.* Gaskell, London, 2002.

Harris G, Bisset J & Johnson R. Food refusal associated with illness. *Child Psychology & Psychiatry Review* 2000; **5**: 148–156. (**This and the Douglas paper above provide a useful framework for assessment and helpful principles guiding behavioural management.**)

Lask B & Bryant-Waugh R, eds. *Anorexia Nervosa and Related Eating Disorders in Childhood and Adolescence*, 2nd edn. Psychology Press, East Sussex, 2000. (**The essential multidisciplinary reference in the field of childhood eating and feeding disorders.**)

Sparen P, Vagero D, Shestov DB *et al.* Long term mortality after severe starvation during the siege of Leningrad: prospective cohort study. *BMJ* 2004; **328**: 11–14.

Stein Z, Susser M, Saengler G & Marolla F. *Famine and Human Development. The Dutch Hunger Winter of 1944–1945.* Oxford University Press, London, 1975.

Further resources

Child Growth Foundation, 2 Mayfield Avenue, Chiswick, London, W4 1PW. Tel. +44 (0)20 8995 0257. Email: info@childgrowthfoundation.org

CHAPTER 13

Eating Disorders in the Family

Jane Morris and Fiona Forbes

OVERVIEW

- A gathering body of evidence supports different patterns of genetic inheritance for obsessive weight losing disorders, such as 'restrictive' anorexia nervosa, and for normal weight bulimic disorders.

- Families where one or more member has an eating disorder will contribute both genetically and environmentally to the climate of response to eating, body weight and shape, and self-control.

- Eating disorders, even if subclinical, can impair fertility and increase the risk of damage to an unborn child. Both pregnancy and labour may be more difficult.

- Up-to-date information should be sought about the relative risks of medication versus untreated disorders during pregnancy and lactation.

- Young mothers who have suffered from eating disorders may need support to learn the skills of healthy, playful toddler feeding.

- Family 'work'—not necessarily involving formal family therapy as such—is the best evidenced treatment for anorexia nervosa.

Genetic inheritance of eating disorders
(Figure 13.1)

There is substantial evidence for predisposing genetic factors in eating disorders—though inheritance does not follow simple patterns. Family studies repeatedly show aggregation of cases within families, and twin studies of both anorexia and bulimia indicate greater concordance for monozygotic than dizygotic twins.

Current research explores particular gene involvement and the hypothesis that separate predispositions to anorexia and bulimia are independently inherited. Sophisticated brain scans examine the forms that genetic predisposition may take in terms of brain structure and function. Scans of patients' family members avoid the confounding effects of starvation on the brain. These reveal unilateral differences in brain function compared with controls.

Psychological research indicates that 'anorexic' families experience high frequencies of perfectionistic and obsessive personality traits. 'Bulimic' families seem more likely to experience depressive and substance misuse difficulties. There is, of course, considerable overlap.

Such research is a considerable way from direct interventions and preventative measures but awareness of predisposing physiology spares families from the guilt and blame often experienced as a result of lay and professional misconceptions, such as the view that 'eating disorders are caused by sexual abuse' or by 'overprotective parents'.

Generational cycles of eating disorders

Since eating disorders occur in a familial environment of increased genetic risk, it becomes difficult to dissect out social and interpersonal causes of disordered eating. All research—and clinical assessment—concerning families needs to take account of the genetic inheritance and thus the likelihood that other family members will be living with at least a predisposition if not with an overt eating disorder. Since 90% of sufferers are women less attention is paid to male family members. Scandinavian work suggests an association with autistic spectrum conditions such as Asperger's syndrome.

Work showing a high incidence of perinatal loss in families of teenagers with anorexia suggests a causative role for pathological grief, but does not control for the possibility that the mothers concerned were themselves of low weight and so more likely to lose a baby. The same study observes that people with anorexia are less likely than controls to have spent a night away from home by age 12 years. This may reflect the personalities of the families concerned rather than be a cause of the disorder. Anorexia research reveals an increase in spring births. This may reflect an increase in summer conceptions in underweight parents who are less fertile when cold weather places extra demands on energy levels.

Eating disorders and pregnancy

Starvation and malnutrition reduce fertility. In Western societies eating disorders are the likeliest causes. The minimum weight needed for menstruation and fertility varies between individuals—ultrasound ovarian scans can help with this. Weight gain can usually

ABC of Eating Disorders. Edited by J. Morris. © 2008 Blackwell Publishing, ISBN: 978-0-7279-1843-7.

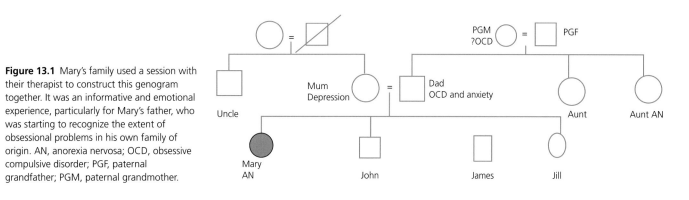

Figure 13.1 Mary's family used a session with their therapist to construct this genogram together. It was an informative and emotional experience, particularly for Mary's father, who was starting to recognize the extent of obsessional problems in his own family of origin. AN, anorexia nervosa; OCD, obsessive compulsive disorder; PGF, paternal grandfather; PGM, paternal grandmother.

restore fertility in the underweight. Young people with anorexia often fear that fertility is irredeemably damaged by the disorder, when in fact with restoration of adequate weight and healthy eating patterns, fertility returns given time. Patients in their 30s with long-standing primary amenorrhoea have been shown to be ovulating normally after weight recovery.

Weight alone is not the whole story. Some women are able to conceive at remarkably low body mass index (BMI) and without having menstruated. This can cause immense distress, but even where there is unhoped-for delight, a partially recovered sufferer may find herself handicapped in both recovery and parenthood compared with someone who is able to take time to prepare for the new roles.

In contrast, normal weight women with bulimia may not conceive. Alternate fasting and bingeing disrupt body rhythms and can be associated with polycystic ovaries. Bulimia can also result in pregnancy occurring despite contraceptive measures if vomiting prevents absorption of pills. The standard combined oral contraceptive pill must remain in the stomach for at least half an hour. It is best to avoid preparations which must be taken at the same time each day. Weight swings make low dose pills unreliable, and can also affect the fit of barrier contraceptives.

Risks of eating disorders and of medication to the unborn child

Failure to gain weight during pregnancy is likely to affect mother even more than child, but to some extent the body compensates by lowering metabolic rate. Self-induced vomiting during pregnancy adds greatly to the risks of foetal loss, need for medical intervention during delivery, and rate of malformations in the neonate. Since study numbers are so far small, cleft lip and palate have been the most common abnormalities observed. Women who had suffered from severe bulimia but managed to refrain from vomiting (though not necessarily from bingeing or fasting) during the pregnancy, had pregnancy outcomes no different from healthy women.

Some women manage to override habitual eating disorder habits at least for the crucial months. As in the case of smoking cessation, some of these maintain their healthier habits, while others relapse after giving birth. Other women struggle in vain against bulimia, particularly if the eating disorder has only just reached medical attention, so that there is little time for cognitive therapy to benefit this pregnancy. In these circumstances it is likely that the risks of prescribing selective serotonin reuptake inhibitors (SSRIs) are

Box 13.1 **Newcastle Teratology Centre Information Service**

For NHS health professionals only
- Tel. 0191 232 1525 (office hours)
- Tel. 0191 282 5944 (urgent enquiries, 17:00–20:00 Monday to Friday)
- Fax. 0191 260 6193 (office hours)
- Poisoning and chemical exposures in pregnancy outside above hours contact NPIS (0844 892 0111), 24 hours

greatly outweighed by potential benefits, and there is considerable experience with fluoxetine both in pregnancy and beyond, including lactation. Paroxetine should be avoided in pregnancy because of an association with fetal abnormalities. If necessary it may be replaced by an alternative antidepressant.

Prescribers can approach the National Teratology Centre in Newcastle for information, advice and interactive support in prescribing for pregnant women (Box 13.1). Details of the pregnancy history are incorporated in the database afterwards, to benefit future prescribing.

Eating disorders and patterns of parenting: the impact of a parent's eating disorder on infant and child

An eating disorder is a potential handicap in the work of parenting (and also on caregiving in other situations—in schools, hospitals and workplaces). Stein *et al.* (1994) highlight the difficulties for mothers with eating disorders feeding their children—overcontrol, lack of playfulness, anxiety, rigidity, obsessional tidiness, lack of respect for child's independence, over- and underfeeding.

Someone with an eating disorder may have had fertility problems, with effects on the perceived fragility of the baby, may be so absorbed by the demands of the eating disorder that s/he has less time and energy for childcare, and may value the child as well as the self so much in terms of body image that other dimensions of life are neglected.

People who have undergone therapy—even if it has not resulted in complete recovery—are often highly sensitive to these dangers, and can guard against the 'temptation' of weight obsession. Sometimes they go too far—encouraging undisciplined eating to avoid over-rigid dieting for their child. Eating disorders often cause sufferers to 'force-feed' their families. This can become abusive, especially if the sufferer is a powerful parental adult.

Scandinavian studies show that young women recovered from anorexia go on to have larger than average families, and recovered patients cite human relationships as the most worthwhile aspect of recovery. They may have extra qualities to bring to parenthood. Sufferers who fail to recover often seem to prefer to withdraw—perhaps reflecting personality as well as a result of long starvation. These people, if they become parents, may find it hard to build up a supportive peer group in which to bring up children, and may be at greater than average risk of postnatal mental illness. Women with bulimia nervosa, particularly in the multi-impulsive spectrum, are also at increased risk of mood disorders, and find that 'dietary chaos' adds an extra burden to the many juggling tasks of modern motherhood.

Primary care professionals—particularly health visitors—have a valuable role if they adopt a compassionate rather than blaming attitude towards such parents at the same time as protecting the children from the eating disorder.

Families in the treatment of eating disorders

Inpatient facilities for management of paediatric eating and feeding disorders are scarce. In any case, the best available evidence supports family involvement in restoration of normal nutrition and eating behaviour. Intensive outpatient or day-patient treatment is ideal, with home visits when possible, so that new skills generalize. Families become understandably frightened and angry when children starve, and high levels of arousal make it even harder to eat. Family education needs to avoid blame but welcome responsibility, acknowledge the seriousness and difficulty of the situation, and teach firmness with calm. It is helpful if carers can understand as accurately as possible what the child feels ('It's not pure naughtiness!') but not let go of the conviction that the symptoms are unacceptable and damaging. Neither collusion nor bullying is as effective in facilitating healthy change as concerned firmness.

The early task of family work is for families and professionals to work behaviourally together towards the child's renutrition and healthy eating behaviour. The therapist incidentally observes family strengths and problems in preparation for the parallel work on underlying difficulties which may block or outlast the feeding work. Communication with schools and any other agencies involved in the child's care is highly desirable. Teachers and youth leaders cannot be expected to supervise meals, but they can set appropriate boundaries on exercise and activity, and they may be able to arrange privacy at mealtimes. Safety issues dictate that schools be aware of physical risks a child may pose. School activity trips may not be safe for low weight children or ritualistic eaters. This is glaringly obvious common sense but easily overlooked by an embarrassed family or a rule-bound school.

Families are now less blamed for eating disorders, and more likely to be regarded as a valuable resource in their management. Indeed, family work is the only well evidence-based intervention for treatment of anorexia nervosa—the National Institute for Clinical Excellence (NICE) guidelines strongly recommend family involvement, particularly for younger patients with anorexia (NICE 2004). The role of family work in bulimia nervosa is less studied. The needs and sufferings of carers—aside from their responsibilities—have only just begun to be acknowledged, and are discussed in Chapter 15.

The Maudsley Hospital family therapy work has been put in manual form, and results replicated in several centres internationally. First the parents are encouraged to mobilize all their skills to prioritize refeeding the emaciated child. Once this is achieved, the family gives back responsibility for eating to the individual and learns to resume normal family life at an age- and stage-appropriate level.

Early trials showed that family therapy gave better results than individual therapy for teenage girls with relatively recent onset anorexia. Further studies found that while traditional 'conjoint' family therapy—if tolerated—gave the best results in terms of family psychological adjustment, weight gain was greater when families were seen separately from the affected patient. Both family interventions were more effective than individual work.

The 'separated family therapy' model involves straightforward supportive psycho-educational counselling, so it can be offered without the need for a trained family therapist. It proved particularly useful where there were high levels of 'expressed emotion' in the families—this expression of negative feeling has been shown to predict relapse in eating disorders even more than in schizophrenia. 'Separated' family work is more practical for older patients who no longer live at home, and whose intense need for privacy mitigates against conjoint work.

More recently, Maudsley professionals have piloted 'multifamily groups', and there are experiments with couple work where one partner has an eating disorder.

Further reading

Bloomfield S, ed. *Eating Disorders: Helping Your Child Recover.* Eating Disorders Association, Norwich, 2006.

Holland AJ, Sicotte N & Treasure JL. Anorexia nervosa: evidence for a genetic basis. *Journal of Psychosomatic Research* 1988; **32**: 561–71.

Lock J, Le Grange D, Agras WS & Dare C. *A Treatment Manual for Anorexia Nervosa: A Family-Based Approach.* Guilford Press, New York, 2001.

NICE. *Eating Disorders: Core Interventions in the Treatment and Management of Anorexia Nervosa, Bulimia Nervosa and Related Eating Disorders.* NICE Clinical Guideline No 9. National Institute for Clinical Excellence, London, 2004: http://www.nice.org.uk

Stein A, Wooley H, Cooper SD & Fairburn CG. An observational study of mothers with eating disorders and their infants. *Journal of Child Psychology & Psychiatry* 1994; **35**: 733–748.

Treasure JL & Russell GFM. Intrauterine growth and neonatal weight gain in babies of women with anorexia nervosa. *BMJ* 1988; **296**: 1038.

CHAPTER 14

Eating Disorders in Boys and Men

Brett McDermott

OVERVIEW

- A small but increasingly recognized proportion of eating disorders sufferers are male, particularly in the younger age groups.
- Gender concerns, homosexuality and the experience of sexual abuse may increase vulnerability to eating disorders in boys even more than in girls and women.
- Presentation in males is more likely to involve preoccupation with muscularity and athletic prowess.
- Until there is more research to guide treatment, assessment and management for male patients should follow the same guidelines as for females, but with consideration given to the benefits of providing a male therapist and avoiding placing a single male patient in an otherwise female group.

Do boys and men get eating disorders?

Published results from population-based, community and clinical studies have reported men and boys are among individuals who experience anorexia and bulimia nervosa, eating disorders not otherwise stated (EDNOS), and limited symptom variants of these presentations. The cited incidence and prevalence rates vary depending on research design, participants and measurement issues. Current evidence suggests the male to female anorexia nervosa prevalence ratio ranges from one to four males per 1000 females with anorexia nervosa; for bulimia nervosa the ratio ranges from 20 to 35 males per 1000 females. In treatment centres there are approximately one male for every 10–20 females. Anecdotal reports suggest the proportion of males is higher in child and adolescent units.

Are there clinical differences in male eating disorder presentations?

Whilst there are currently no definitive studies addressing this issue, results from community studies suggest there are differences in male presentations. Both males and females with eating disorders are over represented in many sporting groups; males are understandably over represented in those male dominated sports that include weight categories such as wrestling and boxing or sports and professions that have clear weight goals such as being a jockey. Boys and men with a homosexual orientation appear more at risk, so too are those who experience some form of abuse. The results of several large population based studies of school students found sexual abuse was a more powerful predicator of eating disorder in boys than girls. Further, boys who experience date rape and date violence were also seen as at risk of developing an eating disorder.

Eating disorders onset may be later in boys than girls given developmental findings that girls have an earlier onset of a desire to be thinner as well as earlier dieting behaviour. These cognitive and behavioural findings are consistent with and likely to be related to the earlier release of adrenal androgens in girls (at approximately 6 years of age versus 8 years in boys) and the earlier release of gonadal hormones (at approximately age 8 years of age versus 10 years in boys). Fear of fatness seems similar in both genders; although fear of fatness in girls may be internally driven, in boys it may be more due to negative peer commentary. One major gender difference is a boy's desire for increased muscularity and a desire to avoid the stigma and bullying associated with being identified by peers as too over- or underweight. Other motivators in boys include the perceived relationship between weight loss and increased sporting achievement; homosexual youth seemed more likely to experience general body dissatisfaction.

Consistent with a desire for muscularity, many males with eating disorders do not display as extreme levels of dieting and food restriction. Boys may preserve protein in their diet. However, as a group boys probably display relatively more excessive exercise as a compensatory behaviour. Indeed for some boys their food intake is within the normal range, it is the calorie losing compensatory behaviour and the motivation for this behaviour that suggests an eating disorder. Bingeing and purging are well described in males. There is also evidence from community research that males abuse steroids to improve muscularity.

Are eating disorders in males the same condition as in females?

It seems that the multifactorial aetiology of eating disorders is similar in males and females. Developmental research, whilst

ABC of Eating Disorders. Edited by J. Morris. © 2008 Blackwell Publishing, ISBN: 978-0-7279-1843-7.

Box 14.1 Boys and men: assessment issues

- Ask all the usual questions!
- Enquire about the individual's motivation for dieting and exercise.
- Body image distortion may be about body 'sculpting'.
- The boy or man with an eating disorder may want to gain weight.
- Ask about steroid abuse.
- Assess the individual's sense of self and sexual orientation.

Box 14.2 Boys and men: treatment issues

- Motivation to change may be eating to promote growth and expected height attainment.
- Self-esteem and identity may be prominent therapy issues.
- Gender issues may be prominent therapy issues.
- Comorbid problems may include depression, post-traumatic stress disorder and the sequelae of child abuse.
- Consider a male therapist.

---

finding higher rates and earlier onset of body dissatisfaction and dieting in girls, nevertheless, reports that boys and adolescent males also desire to be thinner, diet for weight loss and voice body dissatisfaction including shape and weight concerns. In both genders abuse is a risk factor for eating disorders. Both groups experience biological sequelae of malnutrition such as low bone density. Strong evidence for the condition being the same is the substantively elevated risk of eating disorders in the female relatives of males with eating disorders.

Specific assessment issues in boys with suspected eating disorders (Box 14.1)

The clinician should expect a delayed presentation of males with eating disorders given the general perception that eating disorders are conditions experienced only by females. Parent and partner exasperation is also common given their often prolonged journey to find appropriate medical care for boys with eating disorders. Many parents of boys with eating disorders strongly perceive they were not taken seriously by medical and mental health professionals.

When questioning about dietary restriction the clinician should review an average day as they would with female patients. The clinician should not be surprised by less food restriction and maintenance of some food types that may be associated with increased muscularity. When asking about body image distortion, boys will often cite a desire for muscle definition and body sculpting rather than the more frequently cited female concerns of having excessively large thighs, hips and a desire for a more flat abdomen. A boy or young man's fear of fatness may be clearly linked to issues such as bullying. All types of compensatory behaviours should be looked for. Investigations should be similar to those of females presenting for assessment with the obvious exception of malnutrition related amenorrhea. Electrolyte disturbances secondary to purging should be excluded and markers of malnutrition such as age-adjusted body mass index (BMI) and bone density determination should be undertaken. Whilst needing replication, the study of Modan-Moses et al. (2003) reported that malnutrition-related slower growth can be restored with better nutrition, although only 25% of males with eating disorders in their study reached their predicted height. The clinician should also look for comorbid presentations. One could hypothesize that given eating disorders are much more prevalent in females, a male presenting with an eating disorder may have profound issues to do with self-esteem and their sense of identity. Adolescent boys may have specific

conflict around issues of sexual identity. Comorbid depression is likely to be common.

Best practice treatment for males with eating disorders and longer term outcomes (Box 14.2)

The evidence base for interventions with males is poor. Until better evidence is available the recommendations for female patients should be followed. Potential adaptations include psycho-education that a lean body mass does not necessarily equate to nutritional health, and some media depictions of ideal and desirable male bodies may be more due to computer image enhancement or steroid abuse than based in reality. It is likely that discussing identity issues may be essential to therapy, and for boys reintegration into normal schooling may require specific interventions that deal with potential bullying. Some authors suggest that males may not do well in group therapy with female eating disorders patients. They also suggest it may be one place where a male therapist is advantageous. See Andersen and Holman (1997) for further thoughts on therapy with males presenting with eating disorders. As yet there is no specific indication for or against family therapy for younger boys and individual and group therapy for men with eating disorders. It is reasonable that motivational enhancement therapy should be trialled with male presentations. There is very little in the academic literature that differentiates male from female eating disorder outcomes.

Summary

Boys and men can develop eating disorders. Generally the symptoms they experience are similar in range and severity to female presentations. The only caveat being, as a generalization, males have a greater drive for muscularity and therefore present with less food restriction, maintenance of protein intake and more often exercise. The male body ideal, even for a male with an eating disorder, may be for a bigger rather than smaller body. The complications of eating disorders in males are similar to females. Comorbid presentations are similar, albeit the clinician should specifically seek emotional trauma symptoms. It remains difficult to be specific about male-specific management and outcome. Given the current dearth of evidence the eating disorder treatment guidelines for females should be adopted. Self-esteem and identity issues may be relatively more important in therapy.

Further reading

Andersen AA & Holman JE. Males with eating disorders: challenges for treatment and research. *Psychopharmacology Bulletin* 1997; **33**: 391–397.

McDermott BM. Eating disorders in boys. In: Jaffa T & McDermott BM, eds. *Eating Disorders in Children and Adolescents.* Cambridge Child and Adolescent Psychiatry Monograph, Cambridge University Press, Cambridge, 2007: 123–132.

Modan-Moses D, Yaroslavsky A, Novikov I *et al*. Stunting of growth as a major feature of anorexia nervosa in male adolescents. *Pediatrics* 2003; **111**(2): 270–276.

Robb AS & Dadson MJ. Eating disorders in males. *Child and Adolescent Psychiatric Clinics of North America* 2002; **11**: 399–418.

CHAPTER 15

The Sufferer's and Carer's Viewpoint

Jane Morris, Ian MacDonald, Rosemary Stewart,
Grainne Smith and Heather Marrison

OVERVIEW

- Personal accounts of an eating disorder by patients or carers may inspire recovery, teach practical skills for living more healthily—or paradoxically may feed an unhealthy obsession with anorexia rather than with health. Much depends on the stage of recovery of the patient. Most parents are comforted and supported by fellow parents' accounts, but may also be shocked and stressed by unsuspected horrors or by the length of the process.

- Practical and financial support is too easily overlooked. Eating disorders cause both physical and psychological disability but may not be so readily respected by benefits agencies as more clear-cut physical disorders or more feared schizophrenic mental disorders.

- Self-help groups are spoken of with relief and gratitude by both sufferers and their carers.

Sufferers and their lay carers—usually their families—have a great deal to teach professionals about the experiences of eating disorders and their management (Boxes 15.1 & 15.2). Without honest personal accounts of the intrapsychic experience of an eating disorder we are at risk of merely observing physical and behavioural abnormalities and repeatedly fighting these without addressing the feelings, thoughts and assumptions which drive them.

Accounts of the changes needed for recovery and the ways in which these occur can guide effective treatment options. Without carers' perspectives, though, we hear only the blinkered, eating-disordered view of things. The terrible family conflict reported by patients can too easily be blamed for the disorder, but emerges in a new light when we hear of the desperate attempt to keep the patient alive. Carers know the patient intimately enough to be aware of aspects of the illness unnoticed by or withheld from professionals. Professionals who observe family dynamics critically need to know that they too re-enact similar dysfunctional manoeuvres around the sufferer.

ABC of Eating Disorders. Edited by J. Morris. © 2008 Blackwell Publishing,
ISBN: 978-0-7279-1843-7.

Box 15.1 **Case vignette: M's story**

M lost weight in her teens but refused to see doctors. She was always a shy 'loner' who shone academically. Attempts to force her to eat or to take her to counsellors were far more distressing than leaving her alone. When she was stressed she ate even less than usual and took to her bed, so her parents gave up the attempt. She ate little but did not vomit, and her weight stabilized. The family hoped she would 'get over it'. She did well at university and qualified as a scientist, but her weight remained low. She never married, lived alone, and suffered from recurrent episodes of depression.

Box 15.2 **What is recovery?**

One day I was travelling home on the upper deck of a crowded bus. In those days people were allowed to smoke upstairs on buses. All the windows were shut so I was trapped in a stifling smoke-filled atmosphere. I suddenly realized—and it was like a revelation—that I had the option of opening a window to give myself some fresh air. I would never have considered doing something like this for myself before, but I actually did it.

I remember this because it was part of a whole campaign of deliberately taking care of myself, of acknowledging and meeting my own needs—including the need to eat and nourish myself. Anorexia made me deny my own needs but eventually I actually enjoyed defying the anorexia. These days I would be incapable of doing to myself what anorexia used to demand of me.

Personal accounts of coping with an eating disorder: inspiring or unhelpful?

Personal narratives such as Marya Hornbacher's (1998) harrowing *Wasted* or Kate Chisholm's (2002) measured, superbly researched account *Hungry Hell* should be essential reading for professionals working with eating disorders, but families of newly diagnosed sufferers can be plunged into despair if confronted too starkly with harrowing possibilities or the long timescale of recovery. Sufferers themselves can actually relish accounts of eating disordered behaviour in an almost salacious way, rather as they consume diet articles, and 'pro-ana' websites.

The narratives of carers themselves are less likely to be potentially glamourizing, but they too can sometimes discourage families and friends as they confront the stark reality. Unfortunately there is still material available in libraries and on the internet which perpetuates myths that eating disorders are always the result of bad parenting or abuse, so that families who try to inform themselves come to treatment expecting to be blamed.

A helpful approach is for a professional to recommend materials they have used themselves and consider appropriate to the stage of treatment. It is helpful if the material can be discussed and digested later with the professional or in a support group.

Sometimes autobiographical accounts confess that the writing has been part of the author's own therapy, and patients and carers can be encouraged to keep their own diaries and logbooks of recovery, whether for publication or as a personal archive, both to enhance current therapy and for future reference and encouragement.

Buying the book: what works for whom?

Personal narratives often stop frustratingly short of providing effective practical advice on coping and fostering change. 'Self-help' manuals, on the other hand, often provide evidence-based treatment which can bridge the gap between referral and treatment, may be effective when formal therapy fails, and can reinforce the work of therapy or bring extra insights into the work. Wise professionals supply a reading list of recommended texts with which they themselves are familiar, and also cultivate an open, curious relationship so that patients discuss other sources they use.

Chapter 9 has discussed self-help and guided self-help options for sufferers. A growing literature addresses families and carers. Grainne Smith's (2004) *Anorexia and Bulimia Nervosa in the Family* draws on the author's personal experience of caring for an anorexic daughter, and on her subsequent work for the Eating Disorders Association, to present a handbook of factual and practical advice. This ranges from techniques for talking in a 'motivational' way to the sufferer, through lists of helpful resources, contacts and services, to advice on self-care for carers—an aspect often overlooked in many otherwise excellent texts.

Specialist professional teams have produced readable handbooks too. These benefit from broad professional clinical experience and an awareness of the evidence base for treatments, though they lack the poignancy and passion of personal accounts. Lask & Bryant-Waugh offer a thorough account of eating disorders in children and teenagers. Their professional textbook also contains chapters written by a sufferer and a carer. Abigail Natenshon's (1999) self-help workbook for parents is a clear, practical and a useful companion to therapy, and the team (Locke *et al.*) who produced the evidence-based manual on family therapy for anorexia nervosa have recently published a parents' handbook.

Self-help on the internet, and the controversial 'pro-ana' sites

Without guidance it is hard to know what is accurate, what is rubbish, and what is downright dangerous. A fairly safe approach

---

Box 15.3 A bulimia sufferer's story

When I first started dieting and throwing up I felt great—I loved the way I looked and it gave me a lot of confidence for the first time in my life. It didn't last though—the binges started. I was so hungry I had no control whatever—no, I kept just enough control to keep it all secret, but there were times when I stole food and even money to buy chocolate. I was sure people guessed and I absolutely squirmed to think about it. I was a mess physically too—my teeth, my skin, and especially my brain. I had one or two blackouts. It would probably have been a relief if someone had found out and I don't know now why I didn't ask for help sooner. I was so horrified by the amounts I was eating I believed if I stopped vomiting I'd be obese, and at the time I'd rather have died.

Finally I got help because my weight was going up and up anyway and I started to self-harm. I talked to the Samaritans. They put me on to a counsellor who took me through a 'self-help manual'. It helped quite a bit, but what changed everything was getting pregnant—somehow that showed me how important it is to look after your body, and it was actually OK to put on a lot of weight.

---

is to begin with a reputable site, such as those of 'beat', the Eating Disorders Association, on http://www.b-eat.co.uk/Home, or the Royal College of Psychiatrists on http://www.rcpsych.ac.uk/mentalhealthinformation.aspx.

Professionals and parents will find they can easily explore the controversial 'pro-ana' websites. Search engines readily access 'thinspirational' photographs and pathetically obsessed—or perhaps cynically fictitious—messages. The curious surfer is offered shocking insights into the tunnel vision of the anorexic 'cult'—while the eating-disordered initiate is provided with fodder to feed the obsession. It is important to be aware of this 'underworld' so readily available to young people, and to help sufferers find replacement distractions and habits.

Sufferers' views of their eating disorders (Box 15.3)

'Pro-ana' sites may well provide some of the most honest descriptions of how it feels to have an eating disorder. Thinness becomes an almost holy aspiration, and anorexia or bulimia an identity or perhaps a friend ('Ana' or 'Mia'). The Maudsley Hospital's widely used motivational exercises ask patients to write letters addressing their eating disorder first as a friend, then as an enemy. Early in the disorder, the spitefulness of the 'friend' is rarely acknowledged.

Sufferers' views of treatment exude indignation at the experience of coercion, although some patients are generous enough to acknowledge a sense of relief when, at rock-bottom, they were relieved of responsibility for their own survival and nutrition. Many inpatients experiencing behavioural refeeding programmes seem to engage in a 'game' of making it as difficult as possible for staff to increase their weight, using tricks to get rid of food or falsify weight. This oppositional dynamic is demoralizing for staff, and self-destructive once patients are discharged.

The whole point of a genuine recovery it is to take some responsibility for designing and owning the evolution from 'anorexic' to mature individual. Kay Hebourne (personal communication) likens this to a shamanistic journey in which the sufferer emerges from a dark dangerous wilderness into a hitherto unsuspected maturity. The role of the 'elders' is to watch and pray—to oversee the initiation rites and protect the young people from ultimate harm.

The awareness of eating disorders as an 'Achilles' heel' after recovery can be useful part of self-knowledge, allowing a blossoming of compassion for self and others. Sometimes, sadly, recovery from the eating disorder unmasks vulnerability to depression or other difficulties which must then be tackled in their turn, or the discovery that family and friends found it easier to live with an invalid than with a newly recovered assertive personality.

Carers' stories (Boxes 15.4 & 15.5)

Carers' accounts are dominated by the anguished quest for treatment. Paucity of resources is condemned, but ignorance, and failure to recognize the urgent necessity for treatment, cause deep resentment. Primary care professionals emerge badly. Carers feel triply damned—resisted and even vilified by the terrified sufferer, trivialized or blamed by professionals, and regarded askance by a stigmatizing community. There is an enormous temptation to keep the family skeleton in the closet.

When help is finally secured, carers may be too exhausted or resentful to participate. However, those who do manage to mobilize

resources and work collaboratively learn ways of coping which greatly empower the family, and leave each member with greater self-knowledge and awareness of the need for self-care.

Carers speak highly of workshops teaching them how to talk to someone with anorexia—using skills from motivational enhancement. Like professionals they benefit from specific training and from the opportunity to discuss, unload and problem-solve. 'Support' groups are particularly helpful to mothers, but fathers often prefer formal information sessions and active skill training as well as group solidarity.

Practical and financial care for families

Life is expensive when a family member has an eating disorder. Food bills—paradoxically—soar if the sufferer insists on specialized food or if binge–purging is a feature. Heating and transport costs rise in order to protect underweight patients from infection and hypothermia. Hospital visiting drains resources, and if specialist resources are distant from home there may be residential expenses to allow family work. Professionals need to support families' applications for expenses—these are rarely offered as a matter of course, so that the burden of seeking what should be a right adds to the sense of services being grudged and distress invalidated.

Families need assertive encouragement to look after their own physical and mental health. They may need help to withstand 'force-feeding' by the eating disordered patient who cooks for everyone but eats nothing. It can be hard to take a holiday or even a night off, until the patient is well enough to join in. Unless healthy family life continues, though, this precious interpersonal resource will not survive one member's disorder.

Self-help as part of a group or self-help organization (Box 15.6)

Members of the self-help movement could argue that their own support groups more truly deserve the term 'self-help' than

---

Box 15.4 **A carer's story**

My daughter's weight loss was brought to the attention of our GP repeatedly for almost a year before he finally was persuaded to make a referral to a dietician who immediately got back to him to say that our daughter should have been referred long ago for intensive support. Our GP was very alarmed and acted immediately thereafter. He had not thought there was a real problem. He did not recognize the signs. It is certainly true that in that wasted year adverse thought processes, eating habits and exercise excesses became firmly established and the highs provided by undereating were adopted and locked into as a reward for abstinence from food.

Box 15.5 **The stress of caring**

My daughter, Y, was hospitalized and fed by tube. Y is now fully recovered, agrees that this was the right thing to do. But the long-term effects have been worse for me than for her. At the time she fought physically against the feeding and for weeks refused even to see me. She said I had betrayed her. I'm ashamed when I remember it—I didn't cope at all well. I lost my job, and was haunted for months by horrific nightmares. I wasn't much use to Y when she came home, though luckily my parents were around to support us. Eventually I was diagnosed with depression myself and accepted medication and therapy. I found I was very angry with Y, but we're reconciled now.

Box 15.6 **The experience of a self-help group**

My daughter's anorexia showed itself in very rapid weight loss in her first summer vacation from university. Her aunt had suffered from anorexia so she had an idea of what was wrong and was frightened. The worst bit was not knowing where to find help. Our GP advised that a self-help group might encourage her in self-destructive behaviour. For many months she saw a general psychiatrist now and then, but this did not work and she grew worse. It is frightening to find oneself with a professional who seems almost as anxious and uncertain as to how to treat the irrational illness as the sufferer herself, or the carers within the family.

By the time she was referred on to a specialist she had almost given up. The start of her recovery was considerably delayed as time was taken to rebuild trust with the specialist psychiatrist.

Looking back many years later, what helped most was when my daughter was taken seriously, heard and treated as the intelligent human being she is. And the self-help group proved to be one of the most positive and useful points of reference—for our whole family.

therapy produced by professionals and delivered in a manual form. Such groups of course attract those suffering from the severest or most chronic disorders, so accurate evaluation of benefits is difficult. Sufferers and carers new to such groups may be daunted by what they see and hear, although many are simply grateful to find acceptance and understanding at last.

The national Eating Disorders Association and its network of groups

The Eating Disorders Association, now known as 'beat', is a greatly respected British charity. It bridges self-help voluntary, National Health Service (NHS) and private services to offer advice and information. Unlike some militant self-help organizations, it does not promote controversial views and restricts its campaigning to the justifiable demand for improved services and to supporting research. It offers support, training and guidance to self-help groups, publishes both lay and professional periodicals, provides a website and help-lines for sufferers and carers, and has piloted telephone therapy.

Further reading

Bloomfield S. *Eating Disorders: Helping Your Child Recover.* Eating Disorders Association, Norwich, 2006.

Chisholm K. *Hungry Hell: What It's Really Like to Be Anorexic.* Short Books, London, 2002.

Hornbacher M. *Wasted: A Memoir of Anorexia and Bulimia.* HarperFlamingo, New York, 1998.

Langley J. *Boys Get Anorexia Too.* Paul Chapman Publishing, London, 2006.

Natenshon A. *When Your Child has an Eating Disorder.* Jossey-Bass Publishers, San Francisco, 1999.

Smith G. *Anorexia and Bulimia Nervosa in the Family.* John Wiley & Sons, Chichester, 2004.

Treasure J. *Breaking Free from Anorexia Nervosa: A Survival Guide for Families, Friends and Sufferers.* Psychology Press, Hove, East Sussex, 1997.

Treasure J, Smith G & Crane A. *Skills-based Learning for Caring for a Loved One with an Eating Disorder: The New Maudsley Method.* Routledge, London, 2007.

Index